AF842573

HISTOLOGIC DIFFERENTIAL DIAGNOSIS OF SKELETAL LESIONS

HISTOLOGIC DIFFERENTIAL DIAGNOSIS OF SKELETAL LESIONS

Harry A. Schwamm, M.D.
Clinical Professor of Pathology
Department of Pathology
and Orthopedic Surgery
University of Pennsylvania School of Medicine
and
Chairman, Department of Pathology and
Laboratory Medicine
Graduate Hospital
Philadelphia, Pennsylvania

Carl L. Millward, M.D.
Department of Anatomical and
Clinical Pathology
University of California, San Francisco
San Francisco, California

IGAKU-SHOIN 1944

IGAKU-SHOIN New York • Tokyo

Published and distributed by

IGAKU-SHOIN Medical Publishers, Inc.
One Madison Avenue, New York, New York 10010

IGAKU-SHOIN Ltd.,
5-24-3 Hongo, Bunkyo-ku, Tokyo 113-91.

Copyright © 1995 by IGAKU-SHOIN Medical Publishers, Inc.
All rights reserved. No part of this book may be translated or reproduced in any form by print, photo-print, microfilm or any other means without written permission from the publisher.

Library of Congress Cataloging-in-Publication Data

Schwamm, Harry A.
Histological differential diagnosis of skeletal lesions / Harry A. Schwamm, Carl L. Millward.
p. cm.
Includes bibliographical references and index.
ISBN 0-89640-271-1. — ISBN 4-260-14271-2
1. Bones—Histopathology. 2. Pathology, Surgical. I. Millward, Carl L. II. Title.
[DNLM: 1. Bone Diseases—diagnosis. 2. Diagnosis, Differential. WE 225 S398h 1995]
RC930.4.S38 1995
616.7'107583—dc20
DNLM/DLC
for Library of Congress 94-30600
CIP

ISBN: 0-89640-271-1 (New York)
ISBN: 4-260-14271-2 (Tokyo)

Printed and bound in Hong Kong
10 9 8 7 6 5 4 3 2 1

DEDICATION

To Prof. Dr. Erwin Uehlinger (deceased), Chief of the Pathology Institute of the Kantonspital Zurich, and Professor of Pathology at the University of Zurich. An inspirational teacher.

Acknowledgment

The authors gratefully acknowledge the arduous work of Ms. Jacklyn Schacht, who routinely performed miracles with the word processor, and patiently went through endless revisions of the revisions. Our thanks also for the innovative and creative diagrams, the work of Nancy Schwamm.

Preface

In the diagnosis of orthopaedic lesions it is a time honored admonition that preoperative consultation with the surgeon, pathologist, and radiologist is essential for accurate diagnosis. The authorities state that correlation is necessary to avert serious catastrophic mistakes. True enough, but the fact remains it does not always happen; preoperative collaboration and consultation are the exception rather than the rule. From a practical viewpoint, in many hospitals the pathologist is summoned to the operating room suite, performs a frozen section, and consultation with the surgeon occurs at that time, if at all. Preoperative consultation occurs when the surgeon believes there is a problem and seeks advice before surgery.

Most orthopaedic surgeons are familiar with radiographic presentation of lesions in the orthopaedic spectrum. They tend to rely upon the radiograph, and attempt to force the histology into their concept of what the radiograph demonstrates. The confidence with which this radiographically based opinion is expressed by the surgeon can overwhelm the less experienced pathologist.

Self-preservation and reality demand reliance on the morphologic features with which the pathologist is, or can become familiar. Histologic criteria for the diagnosis of bone lesions are present in most cases. While no one is proposing exclusive reliance on histologic features, morphologic analysis can establish a valid differential diagnosis, and thus establish the basis for correlation with the radiograph and discussion of rational therapy. The pathologist must become familiar with histologic criteria, establish confidence in their reliability and reproducibility, and approach the clinician armed with this body of knowledge, ready to collaborate in the management of a patient with an osseous lesion.

Authorities in the field of orthopaedic tumor surgery advise the orthopaedic surgeon not to touch a suspected tumor unless one is ready to complete the entire surgical task. This advice is based not only upon the frequency of inappropriate biopsy, which then endangers the ultimate definitive limb salvage procedure, but also on the undisputed fact that a biopsy commits the surgeon to a specific surgical approach. We believe that the orthopaedic surgeon is a specialist, and that he should be capable of establishing a diagnosis with proper technique even if the ultimate therapy is to be carried out at a center for orthopaedic neoplasia. In this day of electronic communication the orthopaedic physician can consult with the tumor surgeon and discuss the planned approach and preoperative workup prior to biopsy, rather than force the patient (and family) to travel hundreds of miles to an orthopaedic tumor center. The patient is not always willing to travel to such a center for the sake of a biopsy which may prove to be benign; the surgeon may also encounter the lesion unexpectedly. More important, and regardless of where the surgery is carried out, the pathologist does not have this luxury; he or she must be aware of the principles of bone and soft tissue surgery and management, and his or her role in that process. The clinician expects basic understanding of the process on the part of the pathologist during the course of planning the biopsy, adjuvant or neoadjuvant therapy, and ultimate definitive surgery.

This book is intended to familiarize the physician involved in the diagnosis and management of skeletal lesions not only with the process, but also, perhaps more important, with the differential diagnosis. Most short study courses, seminars, and texts solve the most fundamental problem in the title; courses are held and texts are written dealing either with neoplasms of bone, or conversely, non-neoplastic lesions of bone. One of the problems confronting the pathologist and radiologist is precisely that difference; is the lesion neoplastic or not? The superficial histologic similarities of fracture callus and osteoid neoplasia, or the radiographic similarity of Ewing's sarcoma and osteomyelitis may prove to be a significant hurdle in establishing an unequivocal diagnosis. This text attempts to deal with this problem head on. It utilizes the basic histology as the cornerstone on which diagnosis is established. It then uses radiographic and clinical data to support the histologic diagnosis. It is the reverse of what is usually advocated, and of course, it is the reverse of the clinical presentation; the patient comes with a problem, is subjected to diagnostic tests, and ends up with a biopsy and ultimate definitive therapy. For the pathologist, the process starts with the biopsy. The purpose of this text is to demonstrate the intrinsic histologic features which establish a diagnosis and differential diagnosis, the morphologic basis of radiographic diagnosis and correlation, and the pathologist's role in the management options confronting the surgeon, oncologist, and radiation therapist. The text is not designed to be encyclopedic, nor does it attempt to classify all neoplastic or anomalous conditions of the skeleton. The text will not deal with those lesions that are seen primarily in soft tissue, and only incidentally in bone, especially when they do not differ in morphology or management. Thus the angiomatous tumors and anomalies are not considered. Rather, the text attempts to present the common dilemmas confronting the orthopaedic surgeon, radiologist, pathologist, and oncologist and to illustrate an approach to their resolution.

The body of the text is preceded by a short introductory chapter on skeletal growth and development. Structural changes of trauma and remodeling are discussed. A short chapter on the morphologic changes associated with metabolic bone diseases is included.

Contents

Introduction

NORMAL GROWTH AND DEVELOPMENT

The development of the musculoskeletal system follows a pattern of sequential formation, maturation, and removal of mesenchymal tissue. Primitive condensation of mesenchymal tissue results in the formation of precartilage, which is in turn removed and replaced by bone. The bone itself is removed and replaced by more mature bone.

Mesenchymal cells are totipotential. Within certain limits they are able to modulate into any of the skeletal structures in the field in which they are placed. Condensed cells in the center of the limb bud form the precartilage, whereas similar mesenchymal cells near the surface of the limb modulate to form skeletal musculature, tendon, periosteum, blood vessels, and fat. At any age and under appropriate circumstances blastema formation, or reversal to mesenchymal status can occur and the cells regain their ability to transform and modulate into the differentiated structures of the musculoskeletal system.

The Primary Ossification Center

The initial formation of bone consists of a sleeve surrounding the central portion of the cartilage model. This sleeve, collar, or perichondrial ring of Ranvier is formed by direct transition from the mesenchymal connective tissue (periosteum) surrounding the cartilage model. As the cartilage skeleton enlarges, distinct zones are established. The cells in the central portions proliferate, secrete matrix, hypertrophy by absorbing water, and then undergo death of nuclear material. The secreted matrix which is left behind become dehydrated, calcified, and provides the lattice framework on which bone formation occurs (Figures I-1 to I-3).

The dead cartilaginous cell is probably the stimulus which induces vascular invasion from the periosteum. Blood vessels are accompanied by undifferentiated mesenchymal cells capable of forming the differentiated structures of the skeleton, including osteoblasts, osteoclasts, fat cells, vessels, and marrow elements. Osteoid is formed and secreted on the calcified cartilage matrix. The combination of the calcified sleeve bone, calcified cartilage matrix, and primitive bone formed on top of the matrix is known as a primary ossification center. This process extends from the diaphysis towards either metaphysis, and by birth, most of the long bones have been ossified through a major portion of their diaphyseal length.

Secondary Ossification Center

As the epiphyseal cartilage mass increases in size it incorporates adjacent vessels forming cartilage canals in the midst of the cartilage. These cartilage canal vessels do not have an associated capillary network. At specific times, genetically determined, cartilage cells in the secondary ossification center undergo a similar process to that in the primary center, i.e., secretion of matrix, absorption of water and death of cartilage cells, followed by vascular invasion of the cartilage matrix from vessels located at the periphery as well as within the cartilage canals. The secondary ossification thus formed contin-

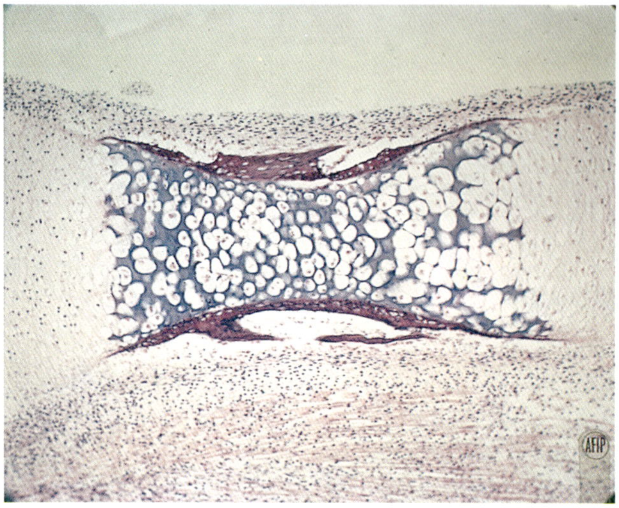

Figure I-1. Endochondral (cartilage model) ossification. The model of the skeleton has been laid down in cartilage. The sleeve of bone is present at the edge, originating from the adjacent periosteum. The underlying cartilage has undergone hypertrophy of the cellular components, and condensation of the matrix. Vascular invasion ensures presence of osteoblasts, osteoclasts, and marrow elements.

ues to enlarge until it is surrounded by a thin rim of cartilage, both on the articular surface and cartilage at the metaphyseal portion separating the epiphysis from the metaphysis. This remaining layer of cartilage is identified as the growth plate, physis, or epiphyseal growth plate (Figure I-4).

Growth Plate

The narrow rim of cartilage that remains between the primary and secondary ossification centers exhibits orderly transition of cartilage to bone and is responsible for growth in length. Distinct zones can be identified: (1) resting; (2) proliferating; (3) hypertrophic; and (4) provisional calcification (Figure I-5).

The most proximal zone of the developing cartilage in the growth plate is the resting zone, in which sparse cartilage cells are embedded in matrix. Isolated cartilage cells are noted to undergo necrosis.

The second zone consists of proliferating cartilage cells, which form well-organized "dinner stacks," actually forming clones and clusters of proliferating cells through mitotic division. The process is three-dimensional, resulting not only in elongation of the columns of cartilage cells, but also in widening of the space occupied by the cellular material.

The territorial (noncellular) cartilage contains copious

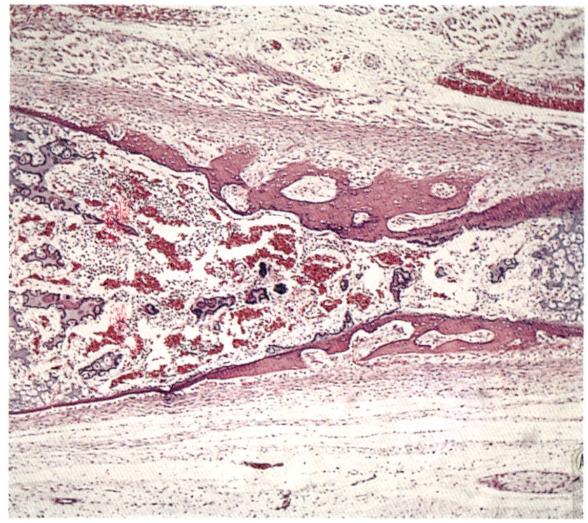

Figure I-2. Endochondral ossification. Extensive vascularization of the marrow cavity, continued thickening of the sleeve of bone by transformation of collagen to bone.

quantities of water which are imbibed into the proliferating cell, causing swelling of the cell. This actually enlarges the physical diameter of the cell, and is responsible for the elongation of cellular material contributing to growth. Growth is a result of hydraulic enlargement of the lacunar space which serves to lift the epiphyseal portion of the bone away from the metaphysis. In the meantime, the dehydrated territorial cartilage calcifies.

One can summarize growth as due to cartilage cells

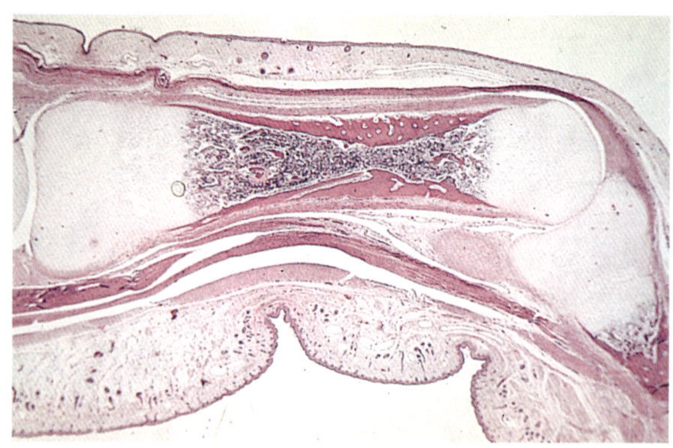

Figure I-3. Endochondral ossification. The diaphysis has been completely replaced by cortical and trabecular bone. This is an example of the "pebble in the pond" phenomenon. Earliest ossification took place at the narrowest point of the diaphysis. At that site the early en coche was formed, and has become progressively thickened. Conversion of cartilage to bone has proceeded toward both metaphyses, growth is somewhat eccentric. At this stage the metaphysis and epiphysis consist of undisturbed cartilage.

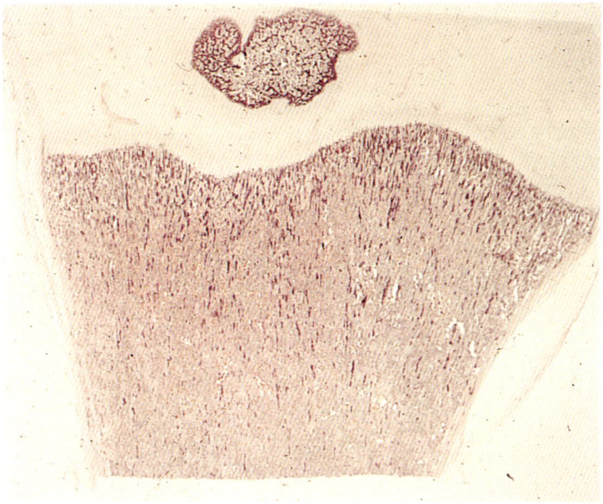

Figure I-4. Secondary ossification formation. In some bones a secondary ossification center is formed, again under genetic control. The earliest manifestation is similar to that in the primary ossification center; there is hypertrophy of cartilage cells, death of nuclear material, invasion by vascular structures, and conversion to bone. The cartilage between the primary and secondary ossification center will be condensed to form the growth plate.

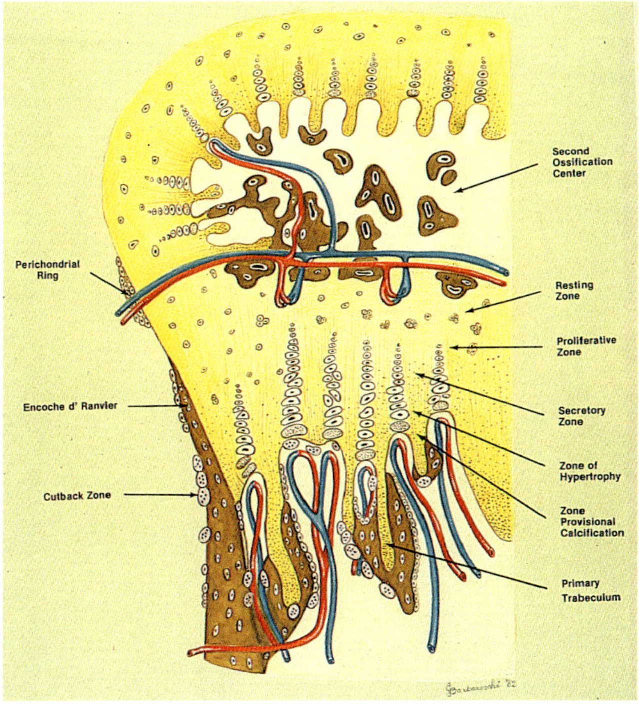

Figure I-5. Schematic diagram of the growth plate exhibiting the resting, proliferative, hypertrophied zone, and zone of provisional calcification. During all this time there is secretory activity on the part of the proliferating cartilage cells.

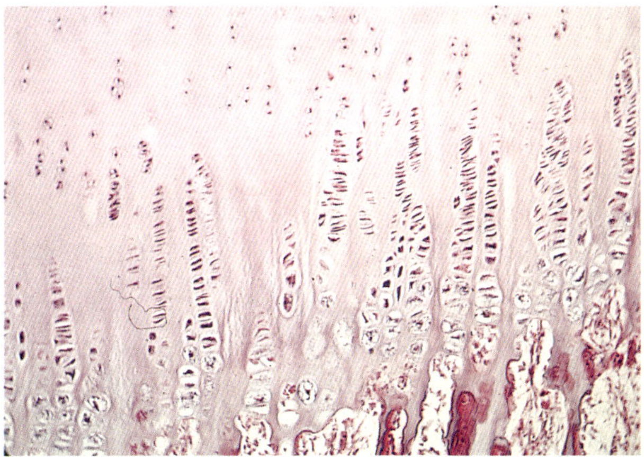

Figure I-6. Note the hydraulic enlargement of the lacunar space of the proliferating cartilage. Growth occurs during this hydraulic lift mechanism. The zone of provisional calcification, provides a firm base on which the entire epiphysis is lifted.

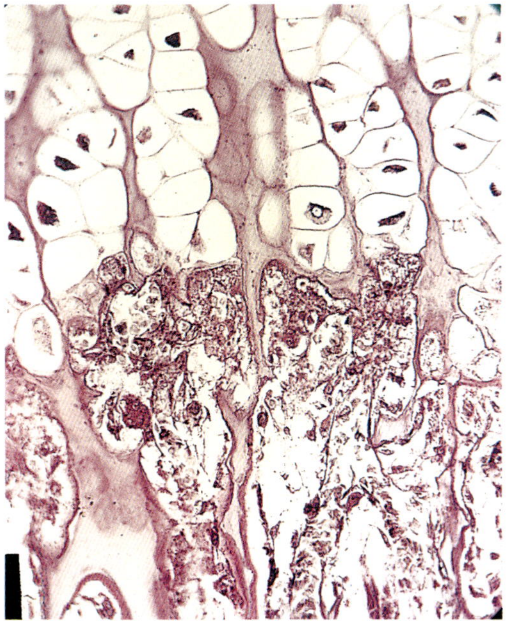

Figure I-7. Higher magnification of vascular fountain at growth plate. Note the enlargement of the cartilage cell, loss of nuclear material, vascular invasion, and coating of the territorial cartilage matrix by a thin rim of osteoid.

Figures I-8, I-9, I-10, I-11. (Schematic diagrams).

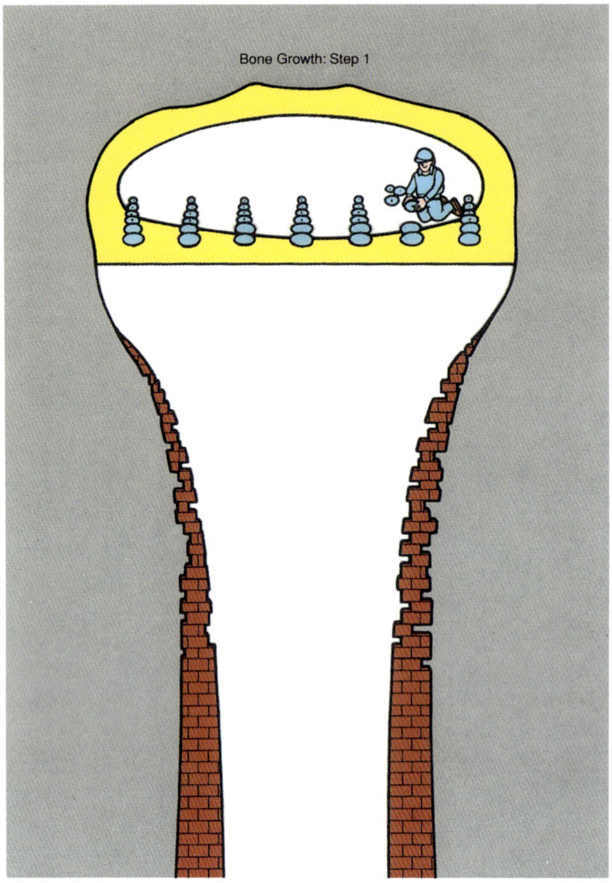

Figure I-8.—bone growth step 1. Cartilage cells are responsible for proliferating and adding to the cellular dimension of the epiphysis. Cellular growth can only occur while the tissue is not calcified. The hypertrophy that occurs provides not only increased longitudinal growth, but also an increase in the diameter of the epiphysis.

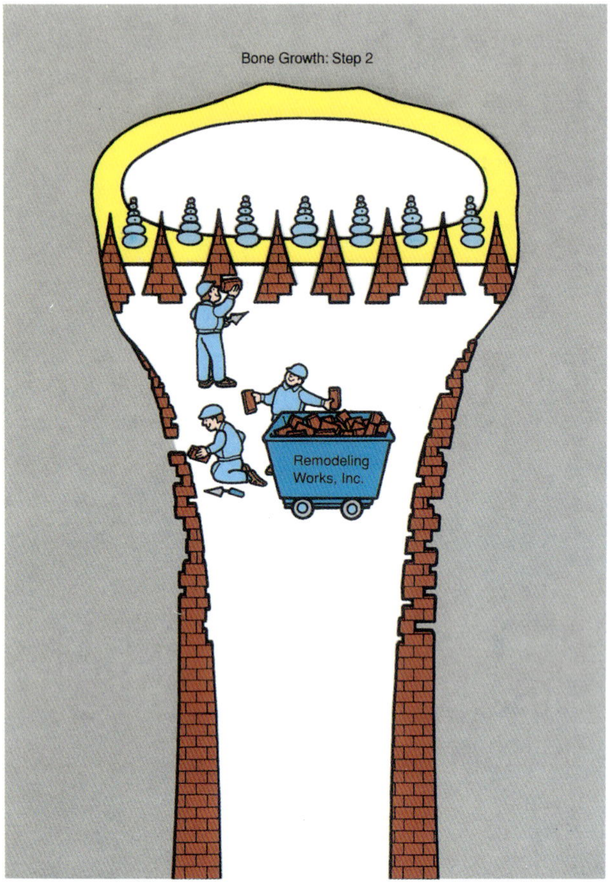

Figure I-9.—bone growth step 2. Formation of the provisional calcification layer and the addition of osteoblastic secretion on the matrix of the cartilage. The formation of this primary trabeculum allows for a solid, wide, horizontally oriented base on which the lifting mechanism of the growth plate can be accomplished.

proliferating, imbibing water (hypertrophy), increasing their size, and therefore their length and the length of the bone. After imbibing water, cartilage cells die. Vascular buds from the metaphysis invade the dead cellular debris, and cellular elements are removed leaving only the calcified cartilage matrix bars projecting into the metaphysis—like docks into a lake. These calcified cartilage matrix bars form the latticework for bone formation, prevent collapse during the death of the hypertrophied cartilage cell, and provide the firm unyielding base on which growth takes place. Osteoblasts, emerging from the vascular bud, form primitive bone on the cartilage framework. Bone is thus formed on a cartilage template. The combination of calcified cartilage bars with primitive bone on the surface constitutes the primary trabeculum (Figures I-6 to I-11).

The cartilage cell is responsible for growth; failure of the cartilage cell to develop results in arrested growth (achondroplasia). Osteoid formation adds to strength and resilience to skeletal structure but is not responsible for growth. The patient with improper osteoid formation does not suffer from short stature, unless there is secondary fracture and condensation (osteogenesis imperfecta).

Osteoclasts are essential to remove the dense primary trabeculae and remodel the bone into its mature dynamically oriented skeletal function. The remodeling pro-

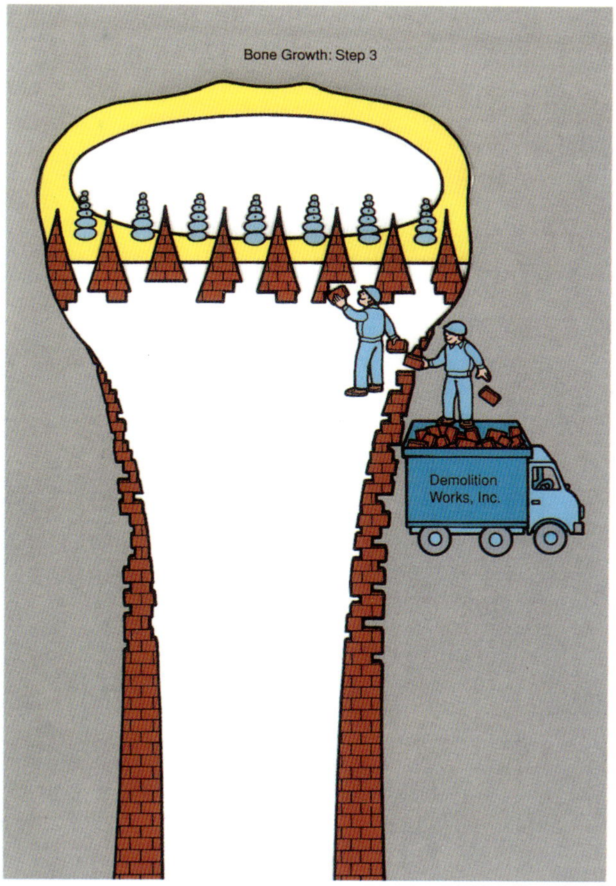

Figure I-10.—bone growth step 3. Extensive remodeling will occur as soon as the lift mechanism has been completed. The wide diameter of the growth plate is remodeled by removal of bone and strengthening of the residual trabeculae. Thus cortical bone is thickened; remaining trabeculae are thickened, but most of the original primary trabeculae are removed.

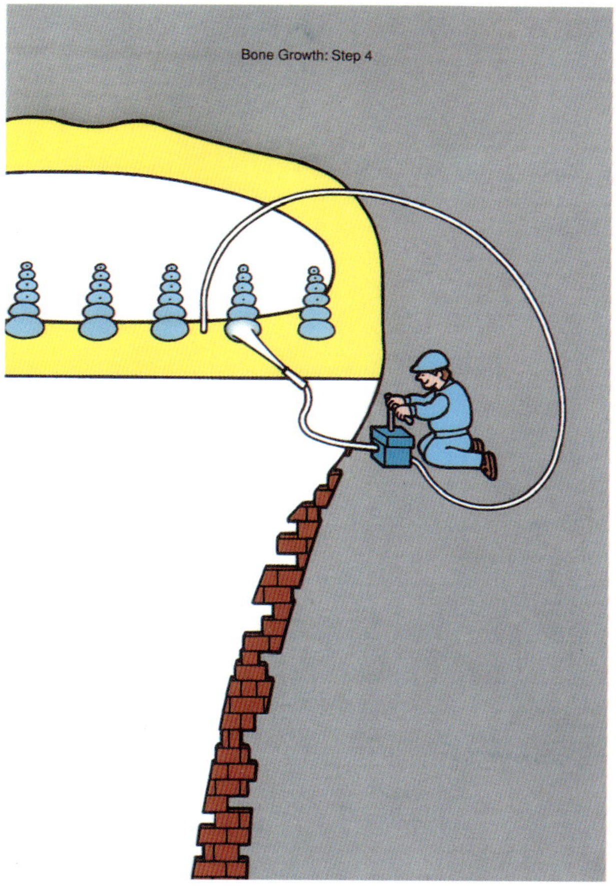

Figure I-11.—bone growth lift mechanism. Actual growth is a function of hydraulic filling of the cartilage lacunar spaces with fluid. The fluid is made available by absorption from edematous matrix. Longitudinal growth of bone is a function of cartilage, not bone. The patient with deficient growth in length has failure of chondrocyte development and function.

cess starts immediately at the growth plate, and osteoclasts are seen removing both calcified cartilage matrix and bone in the immediate subphysis area of the metaphysis (Figures I-12, I-13).

Mature Bone Formation

As the diaphysis elongates, new sleeve bone continues to develop adjacent to the growth plate and remains at the level of the hypertrophied cartilage. This sleeve bone extension, the ring of LaCroix, ensures correct directional growth of cartilage.

Diameter of the growth plate is much wider than that of the diaphysis. Remodeling of the metaphysis is necessary to accomplish the essential reduction in diameter. Funnelization is accomplished by extensive osteoclastic activity. The osteoblastic activity occurs at the same time to strengthen and reinforce the inner surface of the cortical rim. We thus have osteoclastic resorption on the external surface of the bone and appositional new bone formation on the internal surface.

In addition to this remodeling process, growth in width occurs during the transformation from childhood to adulthood. This is essentially a conversion of connective tissue to bone (collagen model bone), and adds 95% of the adult structural bone to any given anatomic site. The conversion process is initiated by the periosteum. The edematous inner layer (cambium) is transformed into bone in a manner very similar to the transformation of cartilage to bone. The zones, because they are somewhat compressed, are not clearly differentiated, but bone formation results in similar fashion by conversion

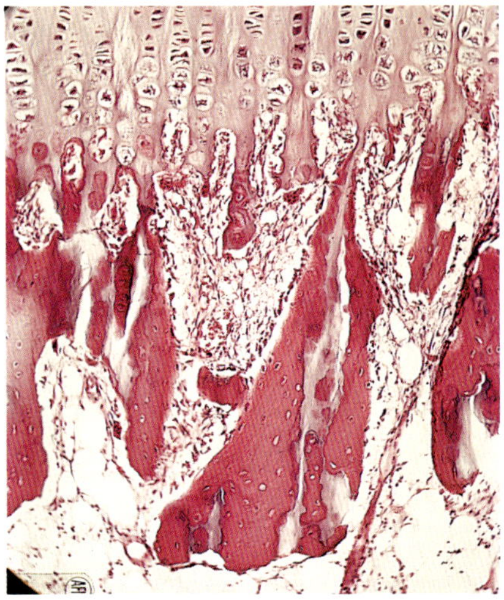

Figure I-12. Remodeling at the growth plate. Note the numerous osteoclasts removing virtually all of the primary trabeculae as soon as they are formed. Instead, approximately 20% of the trabeculae formed are allowed to continue with bone formation, and exhibit the acellular cartilage core (pier in the lake) surrounded by osteoid. This remodeling from a wide base to a tubular structure is consistent with the altered function of the bone in the metaphysis and diaphysis.

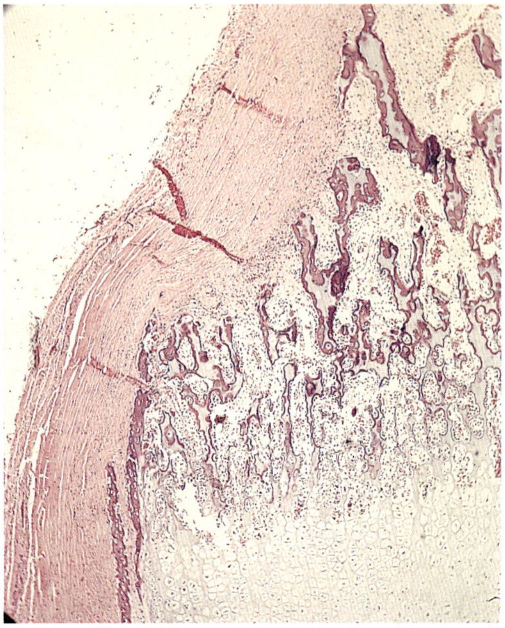

Figure I-13. Lower magnification of the remodeling process, with metaphyseal funnelization. The growth plate is active, and indeed there is extension of the width of the bone by appositional bone formation. A new en coche of Ranvier is formed on the lateral surface near the growth plate. Just beneath the growth plate, extensive osteoclastic activity removes bone to approximately 50% of the diameter of bone at the growth plate. The phenomenon is termed metaphyseal funnelization.

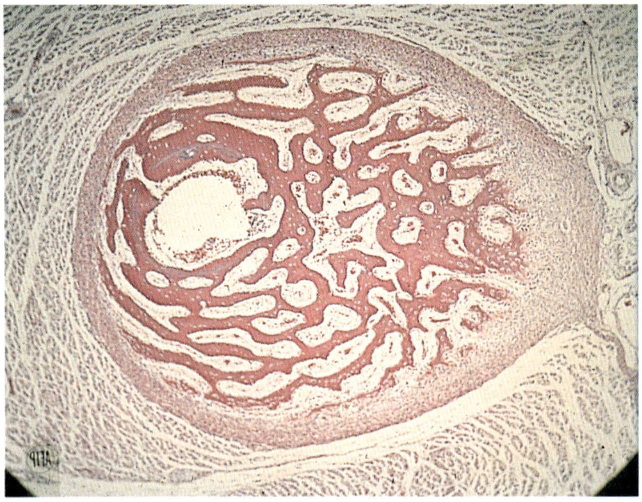

Figure I-14. Periosteal new bone formation adding to the width of bone. The original growth plate and bone formed by the growth plate is located in the cavity at one end of the bone and can be recognized by the residual primary trabeculae. In terms of volume, 70% of the bone is formed directly from periosteum; one can identify an edematous cambium layer and a more dense fibrous layer on the outer surface.

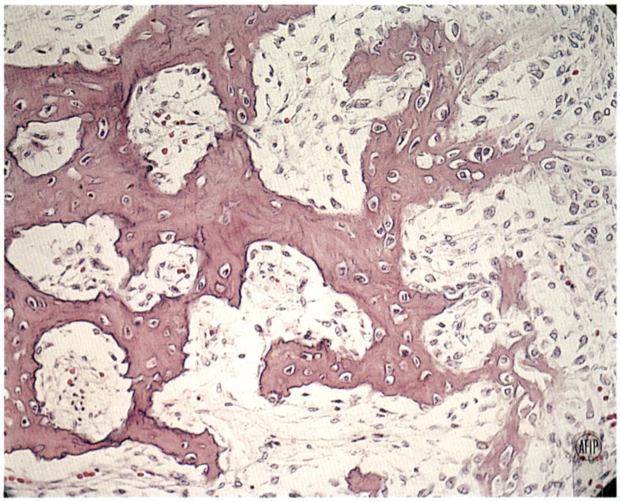

Figure I-15. Higher magnification of the ossification front at the lateral margin of bone. Note the transition from the cambium layer of the periosteum directly into bone. When growth is completed, approximately 99% of the volume of bone formed arises from the periosteum. If the only bone present were that arising at the growth plate, our femurs would be pencils.

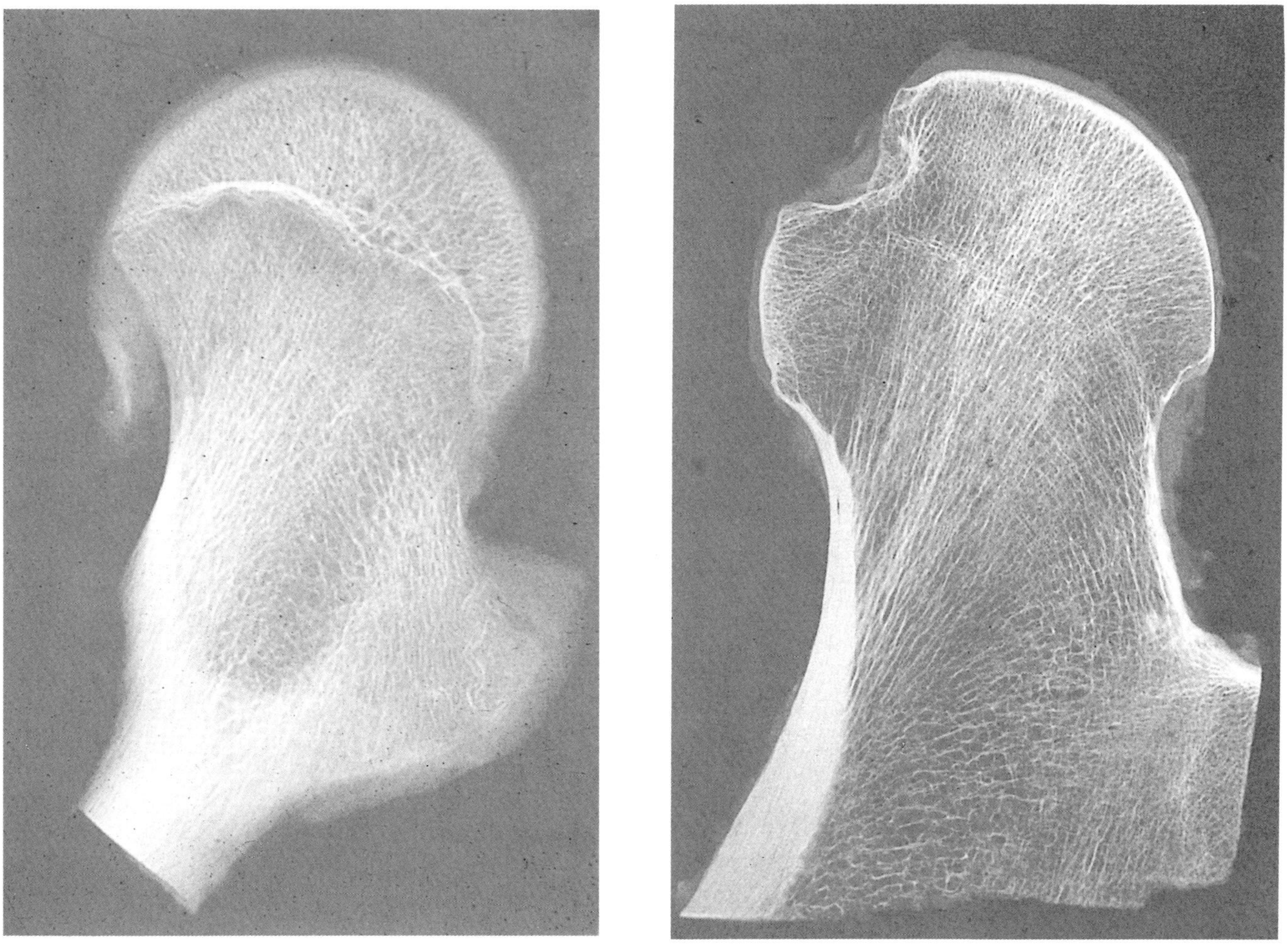

Figure I-16, I-17. Specimen radiographs of the head of the femur, before and after fusion of the growth plate. In the open growth plate, note the trabecular pattern of the epiphysis, distinct from the trabecular pattern of the metaphysis. The two form separate meshworks. After closure of the growth plate the two are remodeled into a single functional unit, following Wolff's law.

of collagen cells, edema of collagen, and transformation to bone. In the adult, when lateral growth is no longer needed, the cambium layer disappears (Figures I-14, I-15).

Internal Remodeling

At a fairly constant age for each bone, cellular replication of growth plate cartilage ceases and the remaining cartilage is completely converted to bone. The growth plate fuses. The trabecular meshwork of the epiphysis is united with the meshwork of the metaphysis, but requires extensive remodeling for realignment of all trabeculae into functional lines of stress (Wolff's law) (Figures I-16, I-17).

Remodeling

As the individual grows and becomes active, bones become subject to muscular stresses during walking, running, standing, and other physical activity, or, in turn, stresses are reduced due to inactivity. Bones adapt to these changing mechanical demands by remodeling, a process that continues throughout life. In cortical bone a cutting cone of osteoclasts appears and proceeds along the course of a haversian canal, producing a resorption cavity. Following behind this cutting cone of osteoclasts, osteoblasts align themselves on the wall of the formed cavity and secrete a cement or reversal line of proteoglycans. Successive relays of osteoblasts produce layers of bone, filling the space from outside to-

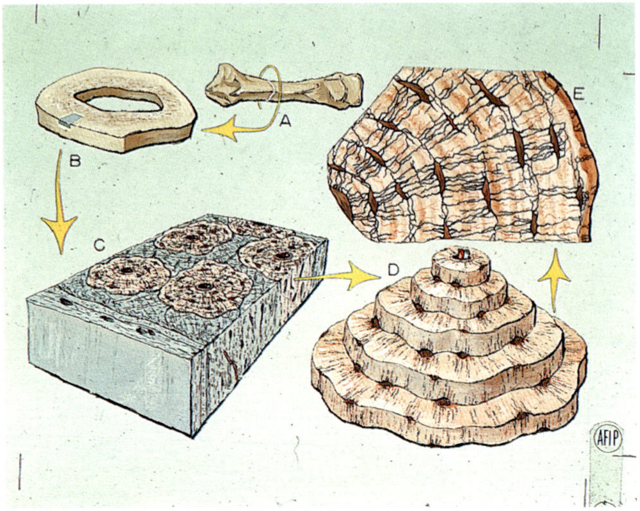

Figure I-18. Schematic model of cortical bone. Cross section of bone designed to illustrate the structure of the osteon. Osteons are found in cortical bone; trabecular bone does not contain osteons.

ward the center, and finally leave a small central canal that contains the vessel (haversian canal). Scattered osteoblasts encase themselves within spaces and become osteocytes. The osteonal system is the basic structural unit of mature cortical bone.

Each osteon has a finite life span. It will vary from 2 to 3 years in a young adult, and may last up to 15 years in an older individual. Remodeling then cuts across previous osteonal deposition, and removes portions of several adjacent osteons. When the cavity is refilled, portions of the initial osteon may remain. After several waves of such activity, small interstitial fragments which are not connected to any haversian system can be identified in cross section. In the older individual, the number of interstitial fragments increases. The age of bone can be approximated by the number of osteonal interstitial fragments as well as the number of rings within the osteon. Younger individuals have more osteonal rings (more active osteoclasts) and fewer interstitial fragments (Figures I-18 to I-22).

Trabecular bone also participates constantly in the remodeling process. Inasmuch as trabecular bone is lamellar (not osteonal), resorption and formation occurs on the surface. The sequence consists of activation of osteoclasts, formation of a Howship lacuna, refill with osteoblastic secretion of osteoid, and subsequent mineralization (see Metabolic Bone Disease, p 14).

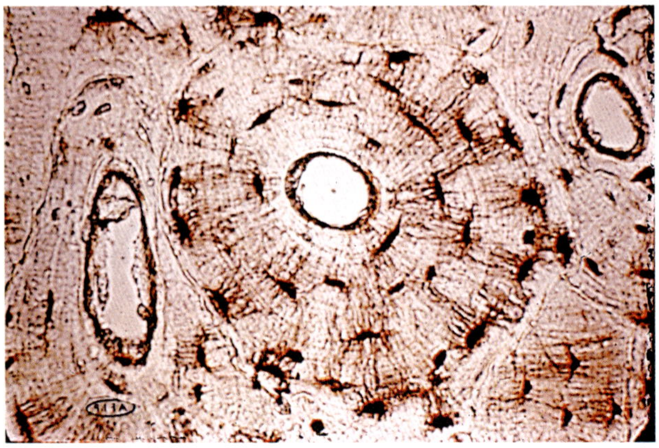

Figure I-19. Cross section of an osteon, exhibiting the centrally located haversian canal, the canaliculi connecting the osteocytic lacunae.

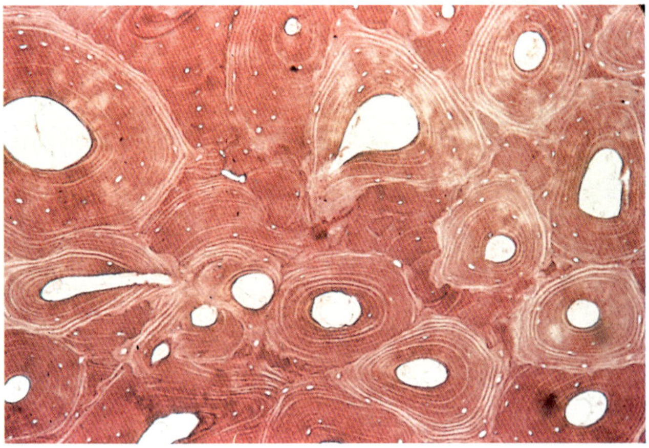

Figure I-20. Cross section of cortical bone exhibiting recently formed osteons, interstitial fragments, and recently formed smaller osteon. The age of an individual can be determined by a cross section of cortical bone. Younger individuals have more energetic osteoclasts, larger cutting cones and therefore larger osteons.

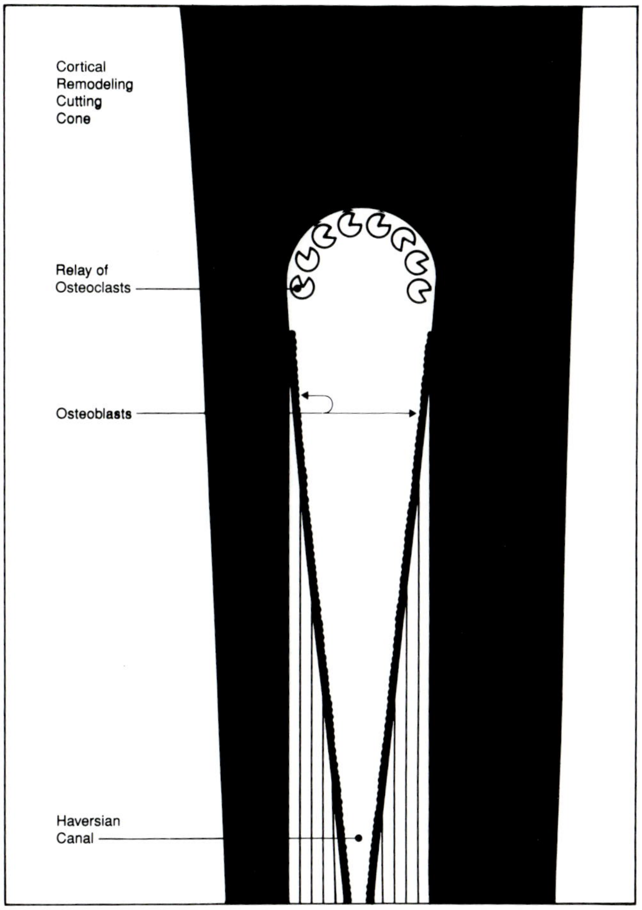

Figure I-21. Diagram of a cutting cone. The remodeling process in cortical bone consists of a relay of osteoclasts digging a tunnel through a preexisting haversian canal or cortical bone. The hole is refilled with osteoblasts, working from the outer surface toward the center of the haversian canal. Successive relays of cutting cones and osteon formation result in the mature osteonal bone of the adult. Excessive activity of this kind with excessive of cutting cones may result in weakening of the cortex prior to the formation of the mature osteon, and can lead to stress reactions and even fracture.

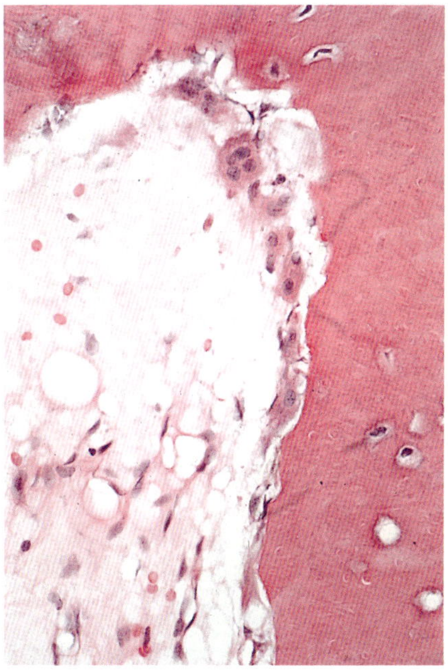

Figure I-22. Cutting cone. Note the relay of osteoclasts followed by cluster of osteoblasts. The cutting cone is the mechanism of cortical bone remodeling, and can occur during fracture, stress reaction, or secondary to infection or tumor. It is simply an indication of active cortical remodeling.

NORMAL GROWTH AND DEVELOPMENT: GLOSSARY

Bone Formation

1. Cartilage model bone = endochondral bone formation = bone preformed in cartilage,
2. Collagen model bone = intramembranous bone formation = bone formed directly from connective tissue, without preexisting cartilage model.

Bone Types

1. Compact (cortex)	Osteonal bone (adult)
2. Cancellous (trabecular)	Lamellar bone (adult)

Ossification Centers

1. Primary	Central, diaphyseal. Precedes formation of secondary ossification center in epiphysis.
2. Secondary	Epiphyseal. Growth plate formed by layer of cartilage between primary and secondary ossification centers.

Growth Plate

1. Resting 2. Proliferating 3. Hypertrophic 4. Provisional calcification. Secretory activity (matrix secretion) throughout proliferative and hypertrophic zone.	Layers of cartilage leading to formation of primary trabeculae

Terms

1. Osteoblasts	Secrete osteoid and encase with matrix to become osteocytes in lacunae. Lacunae are interconnected by canaliculi.
2. Osteoclasts	Remove bone; spaces left after removal are Howship lacunae.
3. Haversian canals	Central canal of osteon: contains blood vessels.
4. Canaliculi	Connect haversian canal to lacunar spaces. Interconnect lacunae.
5. Lacunae	Spaces to enclose osteocytes.
6. Volkmann canals	Lateral connective between haversian system.
7. Cutting cone	Relay of osteoclasts for removal of bone prior to remodeling.
8. Filling cone	Osteoblastic activity to restructure bone after osteoclastic resorption. "Fills in" the cutting cone, from outside toward center.

NORMAL GROWTH AND DEVELOPMENT: GLOSSARY

9. Cambium layer	Prominent edematous periosteal layer seen during growth phase on the lateral surface of bone.
10. Wolff's law	Remodeling of bone is in response to mechanical stress (muscular activity).
11. Ossification groove of Ranvier, surrounded by the perichondral ring of LaCroix	Sleeve of fibrous tissue extending beyond growth plate into the epiphyseal portion of the cartilage model.

Collagen Patterns (under polarized light)

1. Woven bone	
a. Coarse—burlap (rapid) b. Fine—linen (slower)	Earliest bone formation; remodeled to form lamellar bone.
2. Lamellar bone	
a. Circumferential lamellae (lamellar bone)	Without osteons: parallel bands of collagen. Cancellous bone is lamellar, without osteons.
b. Osteons	Basic structural unit of mature fully developed cortical bone with central haversian canal and concentric lamellae surrounding it. 1°, 2°, 3°, and subsequent generations, dependent on remodeling activity.

TRAUMA

Stress Reaction and Stress Fracture

The stress reaction is the result of imbalance between the functional requirements of skeleton and the ability of osteoblasts to meet these requirements. The process reflects normal remodeling of cortical bone. It is initiated by the formation of a cutting cone; relays of osteoclasts resorbing bone in a longitudinal fashion, often along previous Haversian canals. These are followed by osteoblasts lining up along the cavity created by the osteoclast, and filling in the osteon from the outside toward the center. The normal ratio of osteoclasts to osteoblasts is approximately 150 : 1; i.e., 150 osteoblasts are required to equal the activity of a single osteoclast. If osteoclastic resorption of bone is too rapid, i.e., the stimulus for the resorption and remodeling of bone results in excessive osteoclastic activity, numerous resorption cavities and cutting cones are formed, which, at least in the initial stage, results in weakening of the overall bone structure. Osteoblasts simply cannot keep up; there is "unbalanced" remodeling. Under normal circumstances, pain makes the individual realize that the activity is excessive for the structure of the bone. There are circumstances (recruit in the Armed Forces, athlete) under which the activity is maintained despite pain, and under those circumstances actual fracture may result.

The sequential steps in the formation of stress fracture are:

1. The resorption of bone fragments in cortical bone with numerous cutting cones and relays of osteoclasts followed by osteoblasts.
2. Periosteal reaction, occasionally endosteal reaction.
3. Actual fracture.

It is important to realize that the periosteal reaction is simply a scaffold to maintain the functional integrity of cortical bone during the remodeling process. The stress reaction provides the model for all periosteal reactions: in this case increased or excess physiologic activity (unbalanced remodeling), but a tumor or infectious process may well result in resorption of cortical tissue with a similar periosteal reaction.

The periosteal reaction by itself is not an indicator of either reactive or neoplastic activity; it simply represents reaction to weakening of the cortex due to whatever etiology.

A stress reaction or stress fracture under these definitions does not refer to biomechanical abuse. Thus an athlete who continuously pounds a given bone may ultimately fracture the bone; under our definition, this is not a reaction to normal stress, but instead, a reaction to unusual and excessive mechanical abuse which may result in a bona fide fracture. The stress reaction or stress fracture, in the sense that it is used here, refers to basically normal physiological activity requiring extensive remodeling, and will ultimately result in normal bone formation.

Subperiosteal Desmoid

In the growing skeleton the insertion of adductor magnus muscle at the linea aspera of the medial condyle of the femur is a site of fairly frequent erosion, especially in a youngster who is undergoing a growth spurt coupled with increased athletic activity. These lesions characteristically occur in the 13- to 16-year-old individual, and basketball players, cheerleaders, or other youngsters with sport activity. In the growing child the metaphyseal funnelization of the condyle results in fairly rapid reduction of transverse diameter of the bone to approximately 50% of its metaphyseal width at the growth plate. This results in severe and extensive osteoclastic resorption of bone, coupled of necessity with osteoblastic production of new bone at the new cortical margin. Combined with the activity and stresses of the adductor magnus muscle, a temporary deficiency will occur in the quantity and quality of the bone at the medial metaphyseal cortical margin of the femur. Instead of normal bone formation in response to the resorption of bone, the body produces scar tissue. Radiographically this results in a scalloped defect on the external margin of the linea aspera.

This subperiosteal desmoid (Mirra) or cortical desmoid (AFIP) is characterized by dense hyalinized collagen tissue, similar to scar tissue at any other site. The similarity of this collagen fiber to the desmoplastic reaction of the extra-abdominal desmoid has led to the designation "desmoid," but the similarity is superficial, and there is no ominous potential to this lesion. It heals spontaneously with time (Figures I-23, I-24).

Many of the subperiosteal desmoids are asymptomatic, and many of them are bilateral. When they become symptomatic they produce pain, possibly secondary to small avulsion fragments pulled off by the insertion of the adductor. These lesions should be left alone to heal; they are "don't touch" lesions and should not be biopsied. Their rather characteristic typical location on the linea aspera with an eccentric scalloped external defect is diagnostic. The biopsy will only delay healing, and exhibit unremarkable bland fibrous connective tissue, the degree of cellularity depending upon the stage of formation of the desmoid.

On extremely rare occasions such lesions may be seen at other sites, but 99% of all subperiosteal desmoids have been found on the medial aspect of the distal femur.

Fracture and Fracture Healing

Circulatory Phase

When bone is fractured there is reversion to a primitive state and a blastema situation is recreated. At the time of fracture there is injury, which in turn brings about an active circulatory phase. This initial circulatory phase consists of active hyperemia, induced by the neovascularization of the trauma site, with oxygen-rich hyperemia, associated with resorption of bone fragments, closure of the wound, and formation of a blastema, i.e., primary callus. A new field is created, and bone healing will involve all of the mesenchymal structures associated with that field.

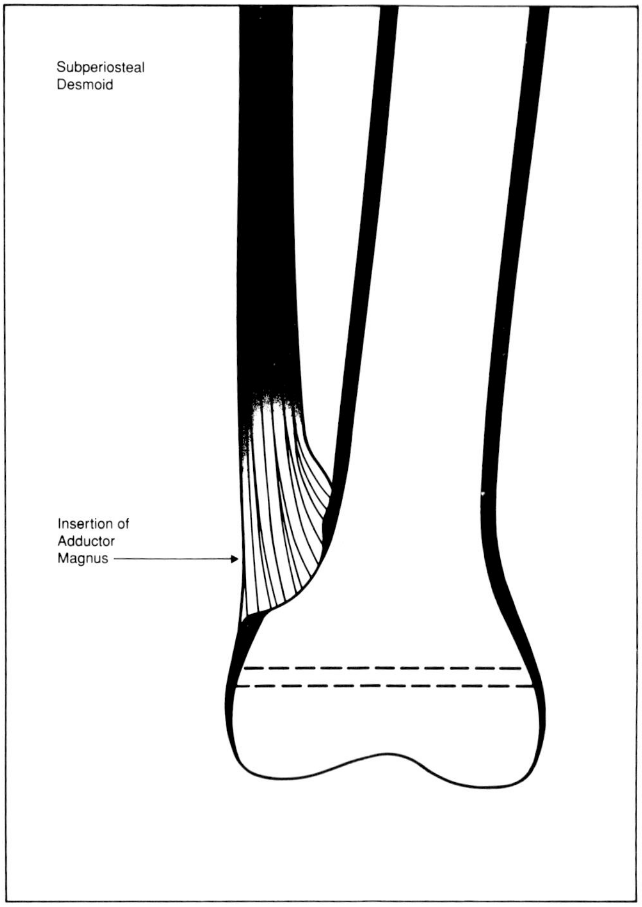

Figure I-23. The subperiosteal desmoid is an example of remodeling gone awry. During the metaphyseal funnelization process, when the diameter of the epiphysis is sharply reduced, the insertion fibers of the adductor magnus may create an additional stimulus for resorption of bone. Under those circumstances the bone may show excessive bone loss characterized by an excavation of the external surface. These lesions exist in the teenager, prior to closure of the growth plate, and should not be biopsied.

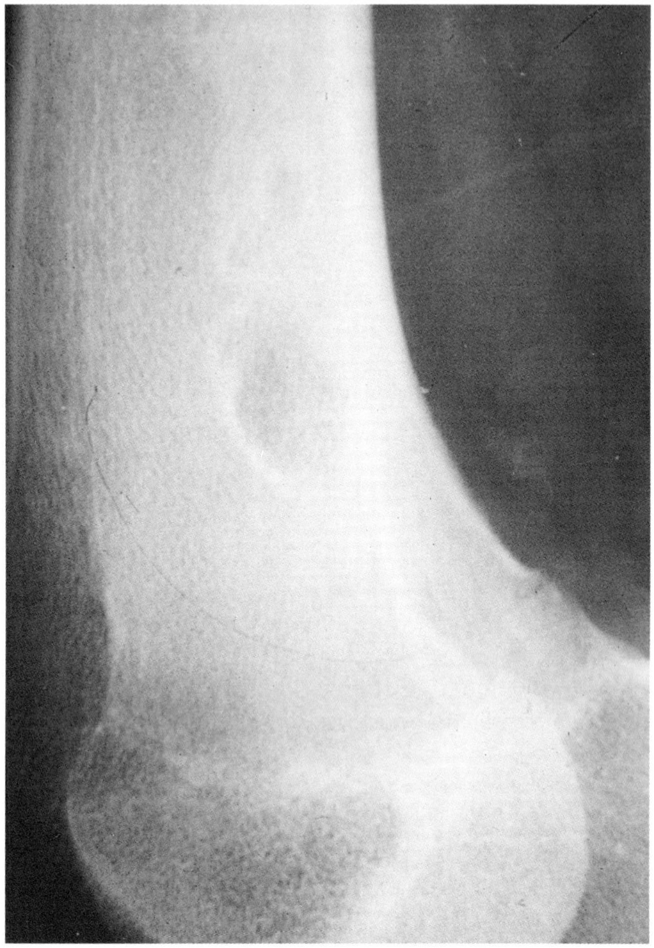

Figure I-24. Subperiosteal desmoid and nonossifying fibroma. The x-ray exhibits the typical external defect on the linea aspera of the medial condyle, but in addition, the patient also has radiographic evidence of a nonossifying fibroma. Both lesions are "don't touch."

In the next phase of fracture healing the hematoma is associated with a proliferation of undifferentiated mesenchymal cells. These originate in the bone, in the associated connective tissue, particularly in the muscle fibers, bone marrow, periosteum, and any other mesenchymal structures involved in the field of the fracture. It is important to realize that fracture healing depends extensively on the vascularization of the primitive callus and the associated mesenchymal elements, particularly the striated muscle. The striated muscle becomes part and parcel of the ultimate callus.

As the healing process continues, bone is resorbed and a vascular spindle is established. As opposed to the initial active hyperemia, this vascular spindle consists of numerous sinusoidal vessels with reduced oxygen tension and slow sluggish blood flow. These factors induce and are associated with osteoblast activity leading to additional bone formation. The primary callus consists of a primitive bone formed by the regenerating mesenchymal elements, including marrow, muscle, periosteum, bone and hematopoietic, and fatty marrow elements.

Metabolic Phase

The metabolic phase consists of a slow healing process. There is reinforcement of the primary callus, clinical union, and conversion of the primary callus to mature callus which effectively immobilizes the two fracture fragments.

Mechanical Phase
The mechanical phase lasts for many years. The united bone fragments are remodeled and adapted to lines of stress.

Clinical healing occurs somewhere in the metabolic phase when the patient is able to ambulate without immobilization and has weight-bearing ability.

The histology of early fracture callus is especially disconcerting to the uninitiated pathologist. It resembles an osteosarcoma. The undifferentiated mesenchymal proliferation is pleomorphic, cellular, and may even show variations in chromatin pattern. However, there should be no abnormal mitotic figures, and the entire spectrum should exhibit a consistent maturation pattern throughout the field. Chondro-osseous bone is a prominent feature of healing fracture (see Figures 3-2, 3-4, p 43).

Complications
Delayed union of fibrous nonunion. Usually occurs in those bones with poor blood supply (lower third of tibia, carpal navicular), bones which have little or no associated muscle. The healing of these fractures requires stimulation of blood supply which can be accomplished by repeated microtraumatization (refracture, electrical stimulation).

Pseudoarthrosis. Created by continued motion without proper immobilization. Requires surgical intervention with removal of abnormal joint cartilage and renewed fracture.

Myositis Ossificans (Heterotopic Ossification)

Myositis ossificans demonstrates the totipotential mesenchymal capability to modulate tissue within the musculoskeletal framework.

The etiology is often associated with blunt trauma, but there are also instances of myositis ossificans associated with neuromuscular and chronic diseases, and those in which no apparent trauma occurs. The disease must be differentiated from myositis ossificans progressiva, a progressive hereditary calcification and ossification of the soft tissues.

The histology exhibits the classical zoning effect which is essential for diagnosis of myositis ossificans. It consists of peripheral maturation of a bone, with sharp demarcation from the surrounding soft tissue. Characteristic zones are formed, consisting of mature bone on the outer surface, immature bone, a fibrous dysplasia-like zone, giant cells, poorly differentiated bone formation simulating osteosarcoma, and finally, in the center of the lesion, an area of simple undifferentiated neoplastic-like blastema tissue. The essential feature in the diagnosis is the peripheral maturation and sharp demarcation from soft tissue as well as the clear dissociation from the bone. In the long run, the lesion matures and forms dense bone.

The lesion may attach to bone at which time the differential diagnosis must include a parosteal osteosarcoma. The radiologist will look for peripheral maturation in myositis ossificans as opposed to the diffuse proliferation at the margin of a parosteal osteosarcoma.

PAGET'S DISEASE OF BONE

Paget's disease of bone is a common, chronic osteolytic and osteosclerotic disease of uncertain etiology. It may involve one or more bones, resulting in pain, skeletal deformities, and, occasionally, sarcomatous transformation. More than 100 years ago, Sir James Paget described the 20-year clinical course and autopsy findings of a man who suffered from an apparently rare, progressively deforming bone disease. It was quickly recognized that the disease as originally described by Paget characterized only the most severely afflicted patients exhibiting extreme clinical involvement. These patients constitute only a small proportion of the total cases. Modern medicine can add little to Paget's century-old insightful and complete description of this previously unrecognized disease, which he termed osteitis deformans.

Histopathology

Paget's disease can be characterized as uncontrolled and irrational remodeling. The disease can be divided into three phases: an active resorptive phase, an active formation phase, and a quiescent inactive phase. Paget's disease is initiated by the replacement of normal marrow with a richly vascular, loose fibrous connective tissue. Isolated clusters of chronic inflammatory cells may be seen. Osteoclasts congregate on the existing bone trabeculae and within the cortex, resulting in the formation of large resorbing fronts. The osteoclasts are morphologically abnormal, many attaining enormous proportions and containing an abundance of nuclei, sometimes in excess of 100 per cell. These striking dimensions and the hypernucleated state account for the designation "killer osteoclast," signifying their overactive functional state. The wave of osteoclastic activity is followed by activation of osteoblasts. The newly formed bone is immature and exhibits a woven pattern when examined by polarized light. Repeated episodes of removal and formation result in innumerable small irregularly shaped bone fragments that appear joined together in a chaotic jigsaw or mosaic pattern, the histological hallmark of Paget's disease. Dark-staining reversal lines or cement lines are formed at the bone interface between these two opposing phases. As the disease progresses, the osteoblastic growth dominates. As excessive formation occurs, bone becomes more compact and dense, but structurally and morphologically this tissue is abnormal. Grossly it resembles the gritty but brittle texture of pumice or lava rock. Radiologically this results in a flocculent, radiopaque deposit, which has been likened to cotton wool. The remaining trabeculae become thicker or more dense, since the width of trabecular spicules oriented along lines of stress are augmented. The cortical bone becomes irregularly thickened as the overall size of the bone increases. The cortical trabecular bone junction at the endosteum becomes indistinct. The fibrous marrow eventually becomes less cellular, osteoclasts disappear, and osteoblasts become less conspicuous. Fat and hematopoietic marrow ultimately replace the fibrous stroma. In this inactive or "burned out" phase, the architecture of the residual bone is markedly altered. Sclerotic bone deposits contain the residual mosaic lines as a sign of the previous pagetoid ebb and flow. It is the characteristic feature of Paget's disease that all three phases may be seen concurrently in an involved bone.

Although the cortical bone may enlarge and expand irregularly, Paget's disease never extends beyond the periosteum. There is no cortical breakthrough, and soft-tissue extension is not seen. **Any evidence of an acute periosteal reaction or soft-tissue mass should suggest the development of a secondary sarcoma.** (See Malignant Transformation of Paget's Disease, p 51).

In the skull, the early lytic stage of the disease can produce extensive areas of sharply defined advancing radiolucency, which may begin in the frontal or occipital areas, resulting in osteoporosis circumscripta cranii. During the sclerotic phase, thickening of the inner and outer tables occurs, with widening of the diploë combined with chaotic osteosclerotic densities due to opaque pumice-like bone deposits resulting in the cotton-wool appearance.

METABOLIC BONE DISEASE

The common denominator in metabolic bone disease is the altered function of osteoblasts, osteoclasts, or abnormal rates of mineralization. In an adult who underwent normal skeletal development, metabolic bone disease will present either with skeletal pain or fracture. Radiographs will demonstrate osteopenia. The clinician must then decide whether the patient has osteoporosis, osteomalacia, an endocrine disorder leading to loss of skeletal mass (hyperparathyroidism), or a neoplastic syndrome associated with loss of bone (multiple myeloma).

It is beyond the scope of this brief outline to delve into the manifold causes of osteoporosis, osteomalacia, or endocrine disorders that lead to those syndromes; or to the biochemical alterations which form the basis of metabolic bone disease. The interested reader is referred to the recent excellent review of metabolic bone disease by Dr. Henry J. Mankin, published in the *Journal of Bone and Joint Surgery*.[1]

It is important to realize that the histologic hallmarks are the same regardless of etiology. Thus osteoporosis will manifest itself either as high turnover osteoporosis, with an increased number of osteoclasts, normal or increased number of osteoblasts, and increased rates of mineralization; or low turnover osteoporosis, with decreased osteoblasts and reduced number of mineralization fronts. Osteomalacia, regardless of etiology, will result in the production of osteoid with defective mineralization. Combinations of osteoporosis and malacia may occur, especially in instances of secondary hyperparathyroidism associated with renal disease (renal osteodystrophy). It is the function of the pathologist to quantitate the morphologic findings, which in turn allows the clinician to evaluate the etiology and therapeutic management of the patient.

Bone matrix is composed of collagen and other noncollagenous proteins and is synthesized and secreted by osteoblasts. In the newly deposited unmineralized state this matrix is termed *osteoid*. The osteoid layer is deposited along the trabecular bone surface and is referred to as the *osteoid seam*.

The mineralization of osteoid occurs in two stages: amorphous calcium–phosphate complexes are deposited into the newly formed osteoid. At a given point in time, after sufficient calcium–phosphate has been deposited in amorphous form, crystalization and transformation to the mature hydroxyapatite crystal occurs. With apology to the extensive research and the individuals involved in this complex problem, the process can be visualized as a supersaturated solution of sugar (amorphous mineralization) which, at increasing concentration, suddenly crystallizes to form rock candy (hydroxyapatite).

Tetracycline has the ability to compete with the amorphous calcium–phosphate complex at the mineralization front. It fluoresces in undecalcified tissue sections. Competitive binding of tetracycline to the mineraliza-

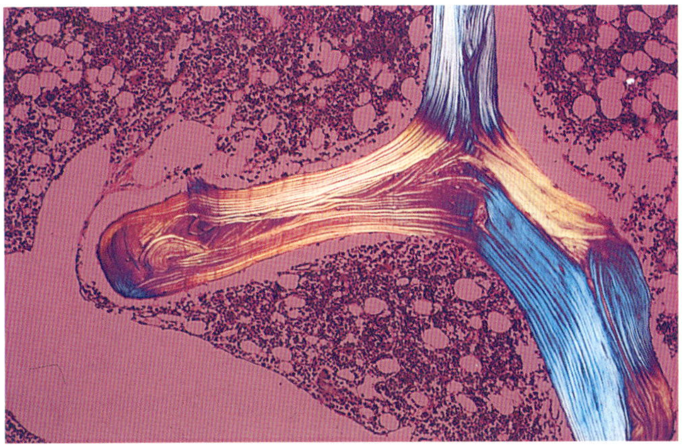

Figure I-25. Trabecular bone under polarized light. Note the concentric lamellae without evidence of osteonal bone formation.

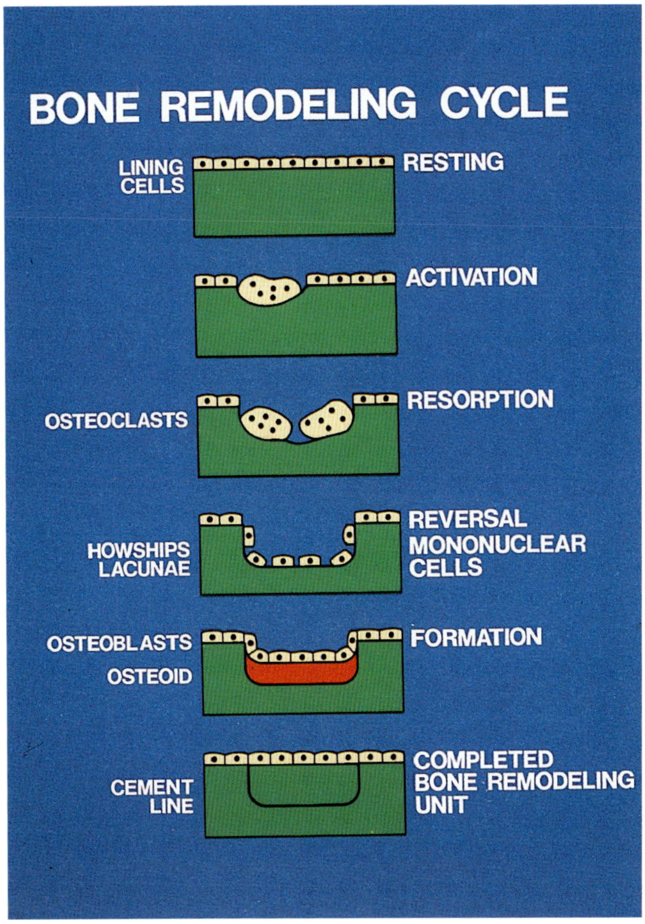

Figure I-27. Bone remodeling cycle. Isolated osteoclasts form Howship lacunae. Reversal occurs with osteoblasts secreting osteoid which ultimately becomes calcified. A reversal line will mark the site of the bone formation.

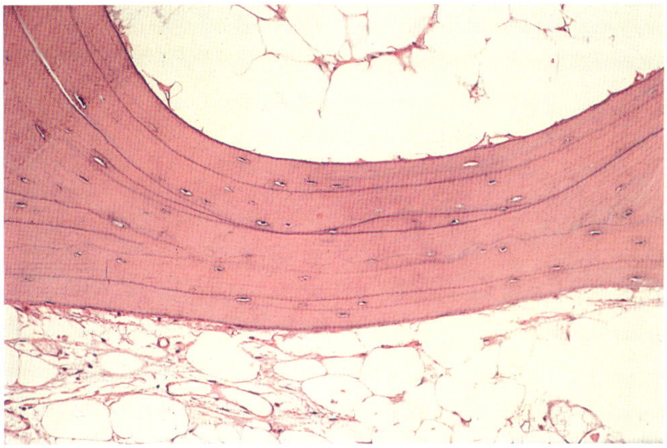

Figure I-26. Trabecular bone with approximately seven reversal lines. The excessive number of reversal lines indicates either appositional bone formation, or possible osteomalacia. No matter what the etiology, seven layers of trabecular bone is not normal, and requires further investigation into the etiology of this appositional bone formation. In this particular case, these trabeculae were found adjacent to a focus of infection.

tion front allows for fluorescent staining with distinctive labels. If tetracycline is administered in two successive doses at 14-day intervals, quantitative assessment of mineralization can be accomplished.

Tetracycline cannot attach itself to the mature crystal. Therefore, tetracycline will only bind to the newly formed amorphous deposits of calcium–phosphate, and not to the hydroxyapatite crystal of mature bone. This distinctive ability of tetracycline allows for determination of rates of calcification. It also allows for qualitative assessment of calcium deposition, and as the patterns demonstrate, can differentiate osteoporosis from osteomalacia (Figures I-25 to I-30).

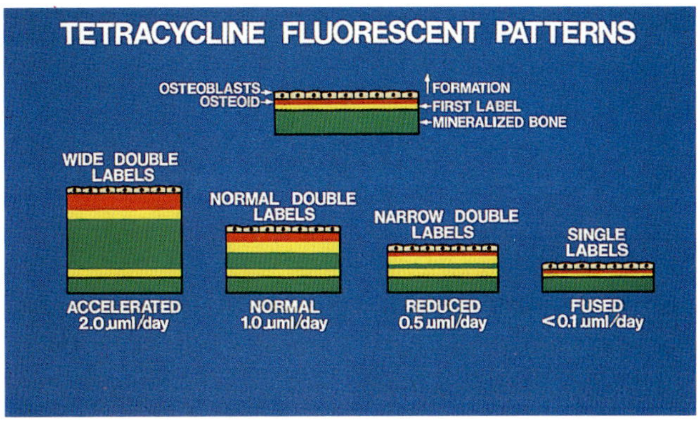

Figure I-28. Tetracycline fluorescent patterns. Tetracycline, by competitively binding at the ossification front, will allow for quantitative and qualitative assessment of calcification.

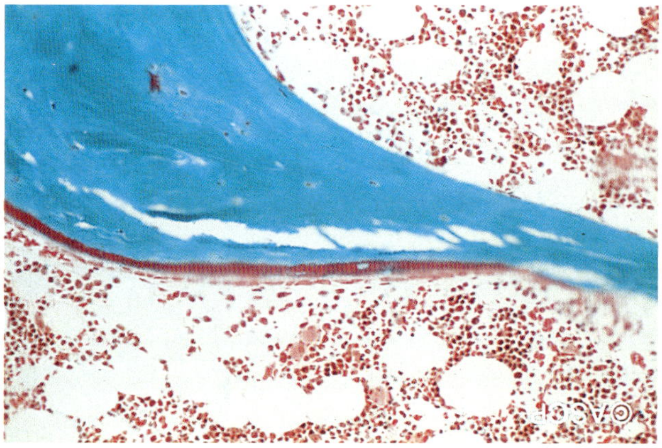

Figure I-29. In undecalcified sections of bone, the hydroxyapatite crystal stains either blue or green with the trichrome stain. Osteoid, with amorphous calcification, stains red. In this particular section an active osteoblastic seam is identified, with a rim of osteoblasts on the surface.

Histopathology of Osteoporosis

The histologic appearance of the osteoporotic syndromes may be classified into two major subgroups, based upon the level of bone remodeling activity (accelerated bone turnover versus reduced bone turnover). Histologic evidence of increased bone resorption and increased bone formation (i.e., accelerated turnover) is termed *active osteoporosis*, while suppressed bone cell activity (i.e., reduced turnover) with minimal bone formation and reduced, but nevertheless, continued bone resorptive activity is referred to as *inactive osteoporosis* (Table I-1).

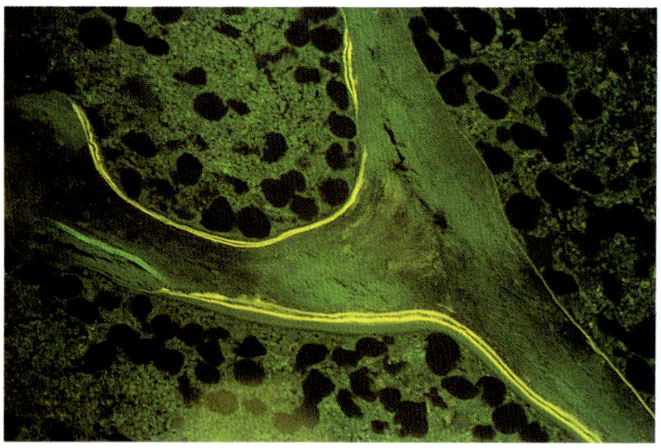

Figure I-30. Tetracycline label of this ossification front will exhibit two distinct labels, indicative of the rate of calcification under normal circumstances. These can be quantified in accordance with the tetracycline fluorescent patterns as illustrated in Figure I-28.

TABLE I-1. Clinical Classification of Osteoporosis

Primary (idiopathic)	*Secondary*
Juvenile	Anticonvulsant drug use
Young men	Glucocorticoid-induced
Senile	Gastrointestinal diseases with minimal malabsorption states
Postmenopausal	Hepatic disease
	Hyperparathyroidism
	Hypercortisolism
	Osteogenesis imperfecta
	Mastocytosis—heparin-induced
	Malignancy
	Starvation, inanition
	Thyrotoxicosis

Active Osteoporosis (High Turnover)

Histologic correlates of increased bone formation include increased quantities of osteoid with an increase in the percentage of the trabecular bone surface lined by osteoid seams. Normally about 20% of the trabeculae are lined by osteoid. The osteoid in turn is of normal width, 12–24 μm in thickness. Because the thickness of osteoid seams may be artifactually augmented by an oblique plane of sectioning, it is often helpful to count the number of lamellae which comprise that seam. Normally an osteoid seam should contain no more than three to four collagen layers. Greater than four collagen layers of lamellae indicates that the seam is abnormally thick (suggesting osteomalacia). The bone surfaces will also contain plump, prominent osteoblasts. Under normal circumstances the fraction of bone surface lined by osteoblasts is equal to that lined by osteoid seams (20%). By tetracycline fluorescence, the bone surfaces will contain double labels (linear bands) of tetracycline. The distance between the double labels should be about 14 μm, reflecting a mineralization rate of about 1 μm/d. As the level of bone turnover increases, the percentage of both the osteoid-covered surfaces and double tetracycline-labeled surfaces increase. The mineralization rate (the distance between the labels) may be increased, as the activity of the individual osteoblasts increases. Increased resorptive activity is manifested as an increase in number of osteoclasts, as well as by the fraction of trabecular bone surface engaged in resorption, resulting in the presence of numerous Howship lacunae. In a normal core biopsy of iliac crest bone there are only 1–2 osteoclasts present in an entire tissue section. More than three osteoclasts per biopsy section is very suggestive

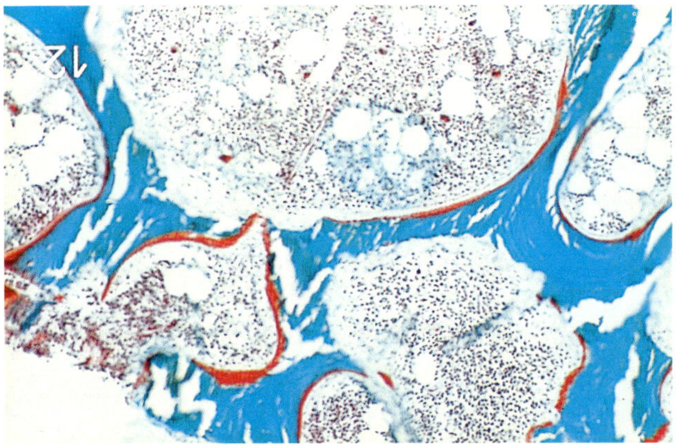

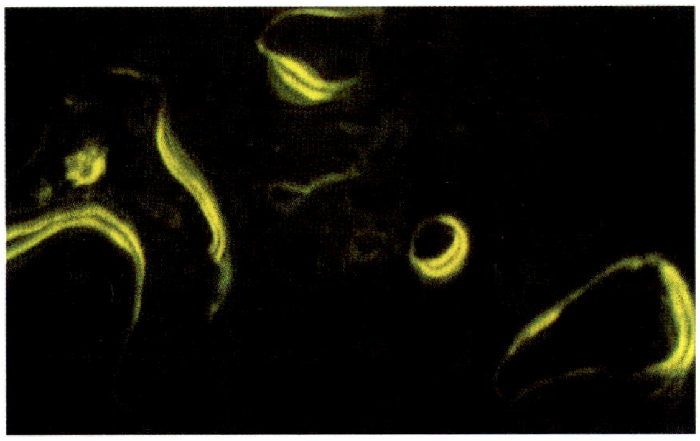

Figure I-31, I-32. High-turnover osteoporosis. The number of trabeculae with osteoid seams is excessive, comprising more than 70% of all identifiable trabeculae in this instance. The osteoid seams are small, indicating normal formation of bone, but at an increased rate. Tetracycline fluorescence of this patient's biopsy will demonstrate an increased number of double labels.

of increased osteoclastic resorption. The clustering of osteoclasts, such that they are found in groups of 2–4 or two of these multinucleated cells within a medium power field (20× objective) is diagnostic of an abnormally high osteoclast number. Normally the trabecular bone surfaces are smooth, and will contain only an occasional resorption bay. These crenated resorption surfaces should occupy less than 5% of the trabecular bone surface (Figures I-31 to I-33).

The presence of peritrabecular fibrous tissue is also diagnostic of rapid bone turnover, and is referred to as *osteitis fibrosa*. Osteitis fibrosa is a generic term, diagnosed by the presence of increased numbers of osteoclasts and peritrabecular fibrous tissue, and is not necessarily pathognomonic of hyperparathyroidism, but may be seen in any state of accelerated turnover.

Skeletal mass is reduced in states of accelerated turnover despite the fact that a normal or even excessive

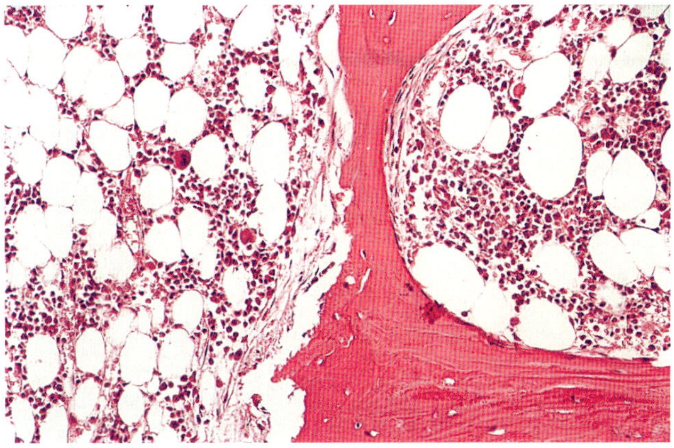

Figure I-33. High-turnover osteoporosis is also characterized by excessive osteoclastic activity in the face of maintained or even excessive osteoblastic activity. Peritrabecular fibrosis, as is seen in this patient's biopsy, is a nonspecific finding, but indicates increased metabolic turnover.

rate of bone formation is seen. Bone formation is exceeded by excessive resorptive activity, resulting in a net loss of bone.

Inactive Osteoporosis (Low Turnover)

Histologically, states of reduced bone turnover show little evidence of either bone formation or bone resorption. Consequently osteoid seams are thin and scanty, osteoblasts are flattened, and osteoclasts are reduced in number. By tetracycline fluorescence, few labels are present, consistent with the amount of osteoid seen by light microscopy. This results in a reduction in the total fraction of trabecular bone containing double labels. The fluorescent tetracycline label patterns reflect reduced osteoblastic activity. As activity decreases, the distance between the labels is also reduced. When the bone formation rate falls to less than 0.5 μm/d, the spatial separation of the dual bands of tetracycline may be impossible, resulting in the fusion or overlap of the two labels to produce one single thin band. In active osteoporosis, the low bone mass is the result of suppressed osteoblastic activity, with a reduced level of bone formation, in the face of a normal or slightly reduced level of bone resorptive activity, again resulting in a net loss of bone tissue (Figure I-34).

Histopathology of Osteomalacia

Abnormal pattern of fluorescent tetracycline label deposition is the hallmark of osteomalacia and represents the morphologic expression of defective mineralization.

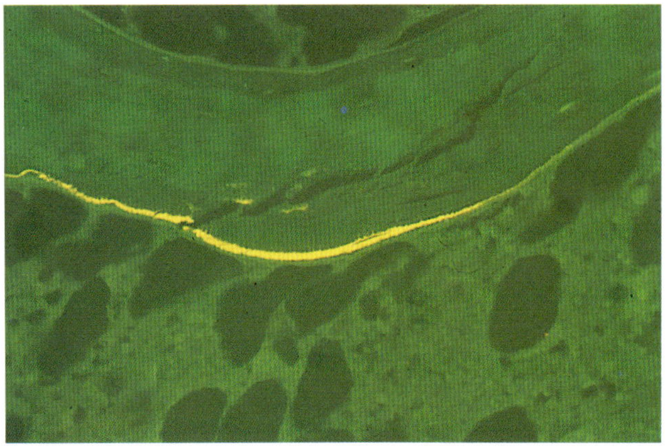

Figure I-34. Low-turnover osteoporosis. No ossification fronts are present. All trabeculae fail to exhibit anything other than resting, quiescent osteoblasts. Tetracycline labeling will exhibit superimposition of two labels to form a single label. These findings are consistent with low-turnover osteoporosis.

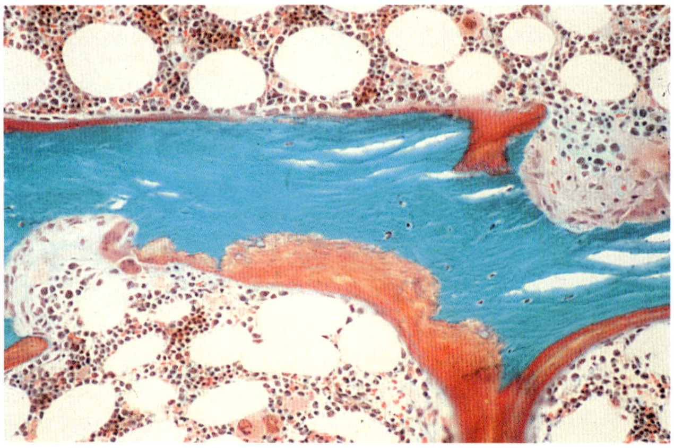

Figure I-36. Osteomalacia. Trichrome staining of the undecalcified section will readily establish that the hydroxyapatite crystal is present in only a small portion of the trabeculum, and that the majority exhibits uncalcified or poorly calcified osteoid.

The amount of tetracycline fluorescence is proportional to the amount of amorphous calcium phosphate deposits in the calcification foci of the osteoid seam. In some cases, osteoid seams are totally deficient in mineral deposits and therefore the osteoid is unable to bind the tetracycline, leading to an absence of fluorescence. A second common abnormal pattern is a diffuse, irregular fluorescence of the entire osteoid seam. This smudging is thought to reflect an accumulation of immature amorphous calcium deposits throughout the osteoid seam without the formation of a discrete mineralization front. Perhaps these initial deposits are unable to mature into mineral crystals. The exposed, persistent nascent deposits thereby permit excessive uptake of tetracycline, resulting in the diffuse fluorescence (Figures I-35 to I-38, Table I-2).

Rickets

Classical rickets is due to vitamin D deficiency in the maturing skeleton, but there are other vitamin D resistant states leading to similar syndromes. Rickets is osteomalacia in a growing child. Vitamin D is required not only for normal calcification for osteoid but also for the maturation sequence of cartilage at the growth plate. In vitamin D deficiency calcification of the cartilage matrix

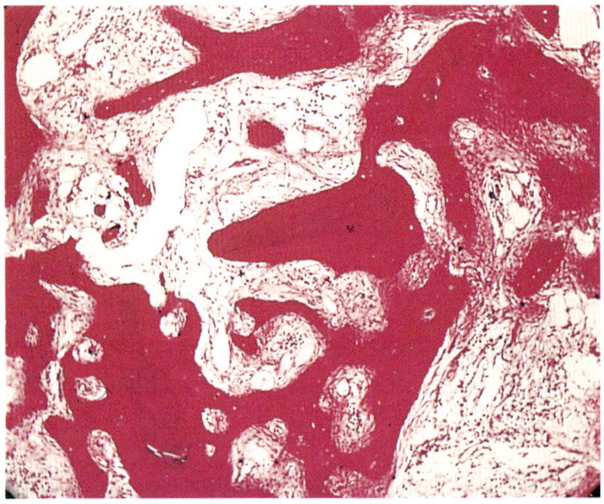

Figure I-35. Osteomalacia. The histologic evidence of osteomalacia without the use of undecalcified biopsy material is often difficult. The biopsy is from a patient with an osteomalacic fracture, but it is difficult to determine whether the material is normally calcified or not.

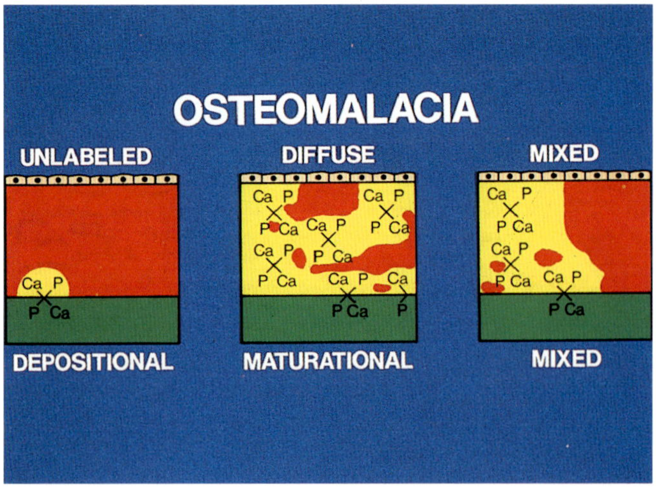

Figure I-37. The calcification pattern of osteomalacia varies, either nonexistent or homogenous smudged pattern, or mixed pattern of both.

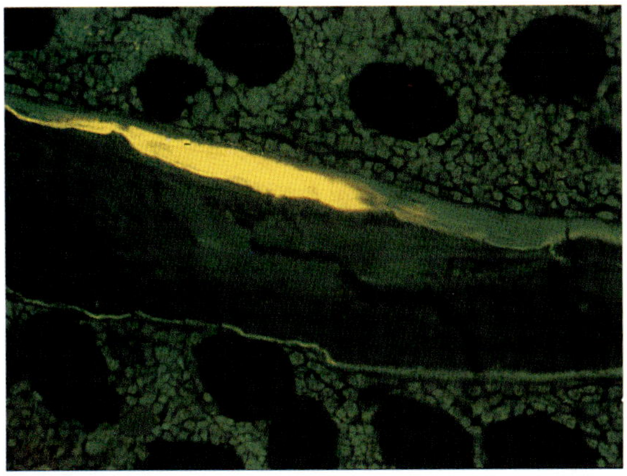

Figure I-38. Tetracycline labeling exhibits a smudged pattern and areas with no staining, consistent with malacia. Patients with combined high-turnover and malacia are usually patients with renal osteodystrophy, and the extent of high-turnover osteoporosis or hyperparathyroidism is useful in determining when additional therapy such as parathyroid extirpation is indicated.

at the growth plate does not occur. It results in uncalcified irregular masses of cartilage at the growth plate, with loss of stability for the growth platform. Osteoclasts cannot resorb uncalcified osteoid or cartilage, therefore the necessary remodeling at the growth plate is inhibited. Radiographically it results in irregular lytic areas of the growth plate (uncalcified cartilage) with lack of metaphyseal funnelization; the "rachitic rosary" of the radiologist (Figures I-39 to I-42). The bone is poorly mineralized, and clinically results in soft malleable bone with bowing. Numerous osteomalacic fractures result (Milkman fractures).

Hyperparathyroidism

In hyperparathyroidism there is increased osteoclastic activity, resulting in maximal resorption of bone. Trabeculae are widened, with central resorption of bone and replacement with fibrous tissue (dissecting osteitis). At the same time, numerous osteoblasts continue to remodel the bone structure. In severe cases, this process results in "trabeculization" of the cortex, with normal osteonal cortical bone replaced by linear trabecular bone.

The histologic changes associated with hyperparathyroidism are the same regardless of whether the process is primary or secondary. The osseous changes are reversible once the primary disease process is corrected, although complete loss of trabeculae cannot be repaired; the remaining trabeculae can be reinforced by appositional bone growth, and become more prominent on radiographs.

Scurvy (Vitamin C Deficiency)

Vitamin C is required to transform chemical collagen to anatomic collagen. Collagen is the basic structure of osteoid, therefore, patients with scurvy demonstrate inability to form osteoid. Calcification is normal.

At the growth plate the absence of osteoid results in persistence of calcified cartilage; radiographically it results in a more prominent density at the growth plate. This calcified cartilage is brittle, and if the patient continues to ambulate, the calcified cartilage layer is fractured and resorbed by osteoclasts. Radiographically the persistence of calcified cartilage involves an increase in radiodensity close to the growth plate, followed by a lytic zone on the metaphyseal side of this increased density, corresponding to the Truemmerfeld zone (zone of debris) in which the calcified cartilage bars collapse and are resorbed by osteoclasts. The normal peripheral rim of bone (en coche) is not formed in a patient with active scurvy. The cartilage will continue to grow, collapse in Truemmerfeld, and, when vitamin C is restored to the diet, calcification of this laterally growing cartilage will result in a radiopaque spur (Pelkan's spur).

The systemic effect of vitamin C deficiency also involves the integrity of all vascular structures. A characteristic feature is subperiosteal hemorrhage with separation of periosteum from the underlying bone. Once

TABLE I-2. Clinical Classification of Osteomalacia

Hypophosphatemic States	*Vitamin D Deficiency—Secondary*	*Hypophosphatasia*	*Chronic Renal Failure—Renal Osteodystrophy*	*Drugs*
X-linked hypophosphatemia (vitamin D resistant rickets)	Hepatobiliary disease			Sodium fluoride toxicity
Sporadic hypophosphatemia	Small bowel disease			Diphosphonate toxicity
Oncogenic osteomalacia	Pancreatic insufficiency			Aluminum deposition
Vitamin D deficiency—primary				

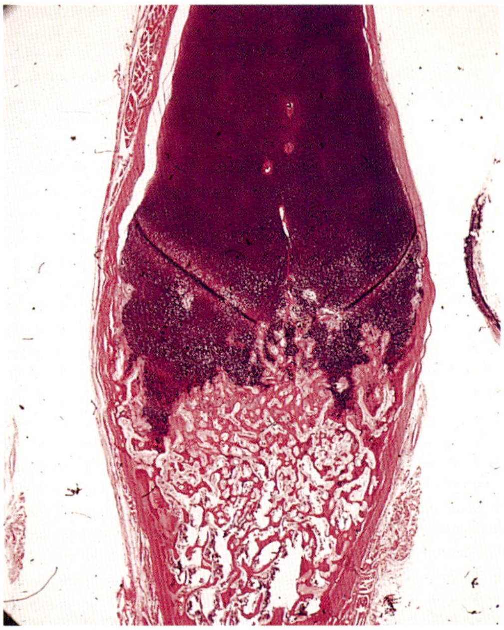

Figure I-39. Rickets. Rickets is osteomalacia in a growing child. The growth plate exhibits irregular masses of cartilage which do not calcify normally, and indeed, do not mature normally causing an irregular maturation front.

vitamin C is restored to the diet, normal osteoid formation is restored, and the separated periosteum grows back to the cortex, mimicking a periosteal reaction.

REFERENCE

1. Mankin HJ: Metabolic bone disease. *JBJS* 76(A):760–788, 1994.

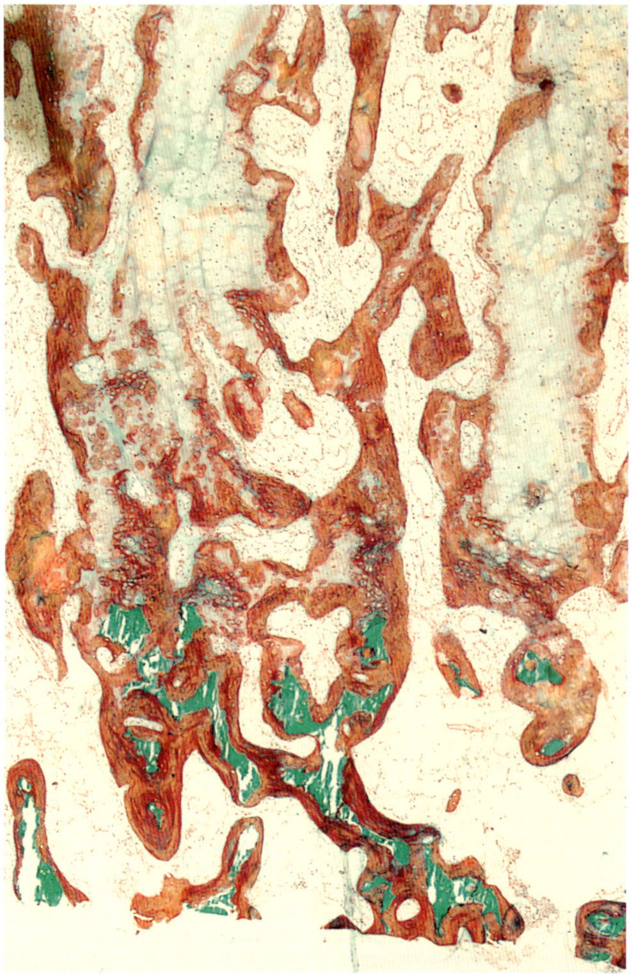

Figure I-40. Rickets. The undecalcified sections exhibit maturing irregular cartilage with only isolated fragments of hydroxyapatite formation (green stain).

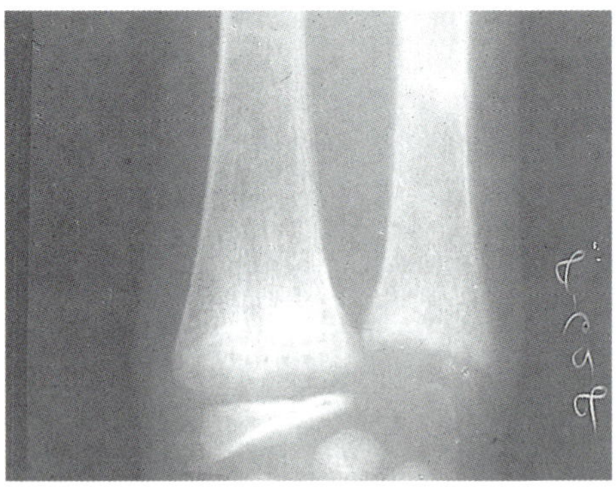

Figure I-41. Rickets. Translating these morphologic findings into radiographs reveals an irregular growth plate, widened, with poor mineralization. Note that the secondary ossification center of the ulna is not formed.

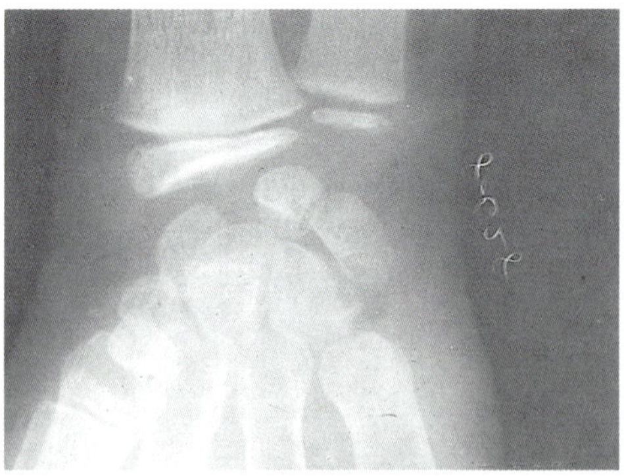

Figure I-42. Rickets. After nutritional support with vitamin D the growth plate resumes normal characteristics, a secondary ossification center is identifiable, and a normal growth plate results.

1

General Principles for the Surgical Pathologist in the Management of Osseous Lesions

The approach to the patient with a suspected pathologic process of bone or soft tissue follows a sequential process which has been described in the orthopaedic literature and should be familiar to the pathologist.[1,2]

The first and single most important diagnostic study remains the standard, plain x-ray film. The characteristics of the lesion, including the extent of bony destruction, the margin of this destructive process, the extent of any periosteal reaction, and the nature of the matrix that fills the destroyed cavity can all be assessed with a plain film. It is extremely rare for a lesion of bone to exist without some alteration of the radiograph, although it must be remembered that at least 30–50% of the bone must be removed before this can appreciated on a plain film.[3] The additional studies that are required to delineate the destructive process are for the purpose of managing the therapeutic approach, but not necessarily to establish the diagnosis. We have attempted to delineate the simple, basic radiographic characteristics of the lesions under discussion with the help of schematic diagrams in the text. It is important for the pathologist to have some acquaintance with the radiographic appearance of every lesion; it takes the place of the gross specimen (see Radiographic Correlation, p 23).

The bone scan is a screening process to establish the presence or absence of additional lesions; it is not necessary to confirm a lesion which is already evident on simple radiographs.

Computerized axial tomography (CAT) scans and magnetic resonance imaging (MRI) are useful in delineating the extent of the lesion and the involvement of adjacent soft tissue, and in establishing feasibility of limb salvage resection.

Chest films are needed to establish the presence or absence of metastatic disease.

These are staging studies, and depending on the surgeon, some or all of these studies are carried out prior to biopsy.

THE BIOPSY

Planning

Once the necessity for tissue diagnosis has been established the surgeon must determine the planned biopsy site. Considerable judgment is required; the biopsy will affect the ultimate surgical procedure. For many years it was thought that the only effective tumor surgery in malignant orthopaedic lesions was a radical excision, i.e., complete ablation of the affected bone to include the more proximal joint. Experience has shown that a wide excision; excision of the tumor, the reactive zone, and portions of the adjacent normal tissue in a given compartment is as effective as radical excision.[1,4–7] The modern "limb salvage" procedure avoids the amputation, and attempts to maintain the normal anatomic function of the affected limb. Obviously, limb salvage procedures can only be accomplished when the tumor can be widely excised, and that, in turn, depends upon the extent of the tumor when it is first discovered. Should the tumor be amenable to limb salvage procedure, the biopsy must be carefully planned.[8] The surgeon should use a small incision; a direct approach to the lesion will minimize contamination across compartments. Drains, when used, should utilize the primary incision or be close to it; local anesthetic should be avoided. The surgeon will thus approach the biopsy with the intent to ultimately extract the biopsy and all drain tracts. In general, the peripheral limbs will undergo a small longitudinal incision so that the entire cutaneous incision can be excised in toto. Unnecessarily wide incisions, horizontal incisions, needle tracts, or infiltration of the tumor by local anesthetic will spread the tumor beyond the original compartment and make a wide excision difficult if not impossible. A carelessly planned biopsy will often lead to local recurrence with possible fatal results for the patient. These considerations appear to be common sense, but it is amazing how many times an inappropriate biopsy will come to the attention of the tumor surgeon who is then confronted with the necessity to perform a radical ablative excision because a limb salvage procedure has been compromised.[2,8]

Once the surgeon has decided to perform a biopsy, the issue of where to biopsy the neoplasm will present itself.

Biopsy Site

If a neoplastic process has extended through the cortex of bone into the adjacent soft tissue, it is often possible to establish a definitive diagnosis with biopsy of the soft tissue component. However, in many instances the soft tissue component is intermingled with the periosteal reaction, and the mixture of the periosteal reaction with or without the neoplastic component is often difficult to interpret and may lead to misleading results. The advantage to the patient of a biopsy restricted to the soft tissue is the avoidance of a fracture. Any biopsy of the cortex of necessity results in fracture, and will require healing. The onset of radiation therapy can therefore be significantly delayed. In most instances, Ewing's sarcoma will have extensive extraosseous spread by the time the tumor comes to the attention of the surgeon, and extraosseous biopsy is certainly sufficient under those circumstances. On the other hand, there are many times when an osteosarcoma is present largely within the medullary cavity; the extension outside the cortex is difficult to interpret, especially with the concurrent microfracture or periosteal reaction. One would therefore prefer a biopsy of the intramedullary component. In lesions not treated with radiation therapy, osteosarcoma for example, the presence of fracture induced by the open biopsy is not a significant factor in management of the patient. Whatever the advantages or disadvantages, it is important for the pathologist to insist upon sufficient adequate diagnostic lesional tissue. Often adequate lesional tissue can only be obtained from within the medullary cavity of a given bone.

The clinicians should attempt to stay away from the site of a pathologic fracture. Early fracture callus can be very misleading, and difficult to differentiate from a neoplastic process.

Closed Biopsy (Needle Biopsy or Aspiration)

There is significant controversy regarding the use of the closed biopsy in the diagnosis of skeletal lesions. We prefer the open biopsy. Needle biopsy does have a role in the diagnosis of numerous lesions, but in skeletal lesions, there are significant disadvantages.

1. Sampling is, at best, marginal. While the presence of a malignant neoplasm can usually be established with a needle biopsy or aspirate, appropriate grading cannot be accomplished. Variability of tumor from field to field can certainly not be ascertained. Needle biopsy may well identify a lesion as a cartilaginous neoplasm, but the grading will depend upon more extensive sampling of the tumor, and that in turn may determine therapy.
2. It is difficult to perform the appropriate immunohistochemical tests, electron microscopy, or genetic markers on the basis of a needle biopsy.
3. A fine needle aspirate can usually only sample the soft tissue component of any given neoplasm. It is difficult to enter the bone with fine needle aspirate, and if one has to resort to a trochar biopsy one increases the risk of needle tract contamination as well as pathologic fracture.
4. In the best of hands, diagnostic lesional tissue is obtained only 66–80% of the time.[9]
5. One should not forget that despite statements to

the contrary, a needle tract is a potential source of contamination.[10] Any ultimate definitive surgical procedure must encompass the entire biopsy tract, including all needle tracts as well as local anesthetic needle tracts. Failure to do so leads to local recurrence.

There are times when needle aspiration or biopsy is appropriate. Soft tissue tumors are easily approached with needle biopsy, as is the suspected local recurrence of a previously diagnosed primary neoplasm. A patient with suspected myeloma or other hematopoietic disorder is a fitting candidate. There are times when the radiographic and clinical evidence points to osteosarcoma; radical surgery is the only option, and the evidence is so strong confirmation is more a matter of record than a problem in diagnosis. Under those circumstances a needle biopsy may be appropriate. There are anatomic locations that make open biopsies difficult; vertebral body biopsies come to mind, and under those circumstances a needle biopsy is certainly appropriate. There is no argument with the fact that a needle biopsy saves general anesthesia, is less costly, and does not require hospitalization. In the final analysis needle aspiration or biopsy depends on the confidence of the pathologist in interpreting scattered cells.

The pathologist, who bears the ultimate responsibility for the correct diagnosis (and subsequent therapy), should not hesitate to demand the optimal opportunity to establish the correct diagnosis. All other factors being equal, in our practice we prefer open biopsy with adequate tissue sampling as determined on frozen section.

Diagnosis

Once the biopsy is performed the surgeon expects the pathologist to answer the following questions:

1. Is the tissue obtained representative of the lesion?
2. Is there enough to establish a diagnosis?
3. Is the proposed diagnosis consistent with the radiographic appearance?

Frozen Section

Always! The role of the frozen section is to determine whether there is (a) representative sampling of the lesional tissue, and (b) maintained viability.

One should never shy away from a frozen section—after all, that's what surgical pathology is all about. The preparation of a frozen section of intraosseous tissue is usually not difficult, and despite the presence of small calcified particles there is usually enough malleable tissue to allow the preparation of material that can be readily sectioned and interpreted (Figure 1-1). A patient who is undergoing a diagnostic biopsy for a suspected pathologic process always requires a frozen section. If the lesion has benign radiographic characteristics and the surgeon is convinced that the process can be managed with an intralesional excision, i.e., curettage, frozen section will serve to confirm that impression and allow the surgeon to continue with planned therapy. In case of a malignant tumor, the purpose of the frozen section is not necessarily to establish a diagnosis, but rather: (1) to ensure that the tissue removed is viable, and (2) that there is sufficient tissue available to establish a definite pathologic diagnosis on permanent sections. Necrotic tissue is often present within the lesion, and if the biopsy only produces hyalinized or necrotic tissue, it is of no use to the pathologist (Figure 1-2). If not recognized at the time of biopsy, it subjects the patient to an unnecessary second procedure and anesthesia. Therefore, frozen section is mandatory; the purpose is to establish presence of adequate viable tissue for diagnostic purposes, but it must be stressed that the definitive diagnosis should be made only after the study has been completed, including immunohistochemical stains, electron microscopy, genetic markers, and other techniques.

Adjuvant chemotherapy, radiation therapy, antibiotic therapy, additional surgery, or any combination of those can wait 24 to 48 hours or even longer without serious harm to the patient. There is time for thoughtful complete study of the lesion prior to rendering diagnoses.

Radiologic Correlation

In attempting to answer the question of whether the proposed diagnosis is consistent with the radiographic appearance, one must obviously have some clue as to the radiographic appearance of bone lesions. The radiologist attempts to define the bone lesion on the basis of three distinct patterns:[11–13]

1. *Bone destruction.* If destruction is rapid, the margins of the lesion will be indistinct and the radiologist speaks of moth-eaten or permeative destructive patterns. These patterns imply a fast rapidly destroying process, and can either be a rapidly developing tumor, or an inflammatory process with rapid progression. If the lesion is slow growing, the radiographic margins will be distinct, sharp, and there may even be a rim of reactive bone at the edge of the lesion. Osteoclasts work rapidly; visible bone removal can occur within days. Bone formation is a relatively slow phenomenon, takes weeks to become apparent on a radiograph, and therefore a reactive rim of bone implies a slow growing (i.e., benign) process (Figures 1-3 to 1-12).

2. *Periosteal reaction.* A periosteal reaction is a re-

X-RAY MARGINS

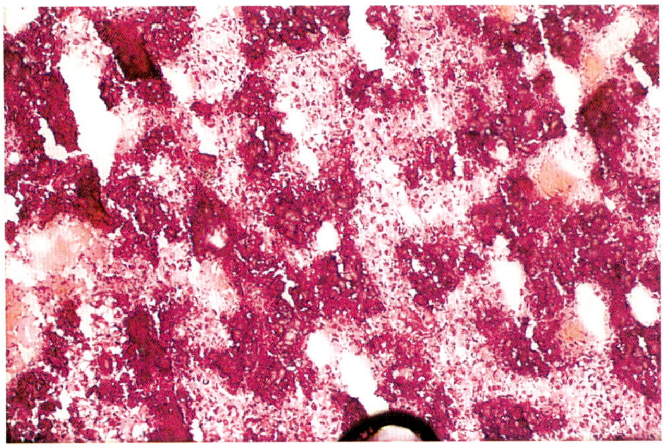

Figure 1-1. Frozen section of osteosarcoma, osteoblastoma-like. Despite heavily calcified material, a frozen section can be performed, and exhibits what is obviously tumor bone and tumor cells. This is an adequate specimen because it identifies lesional tissue. The precise nature of the tumor should be determined after permanent sections are obtained.

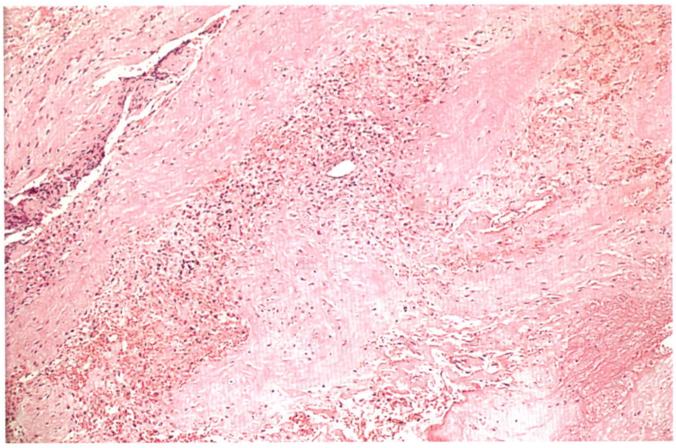

Figure 1-2. Biopsy of suspected sarcoma. The histologic picture exhibits partially necrotic tissue without identifiable diagnostic elements. On frozen section this is an unsatisfactory specimen. Additional biopsy material is mandatory. A second biopsy confirmed the presence of osteosarcoma.

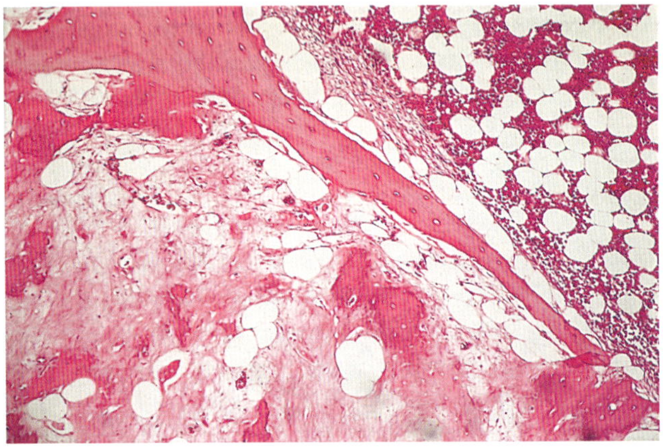

Figure 1-3. X-ray margins: geographic. A rim of trabecular bone surrounding a proliferation of cartilaginous and osseous elements; the nature of the process is slow growing, due to the rim of adult bone encompassing the lesion and the presence of unremarkable marrow on the opposite side of the lesion. The radiograph of this process should show a sharply defined geographic margin.

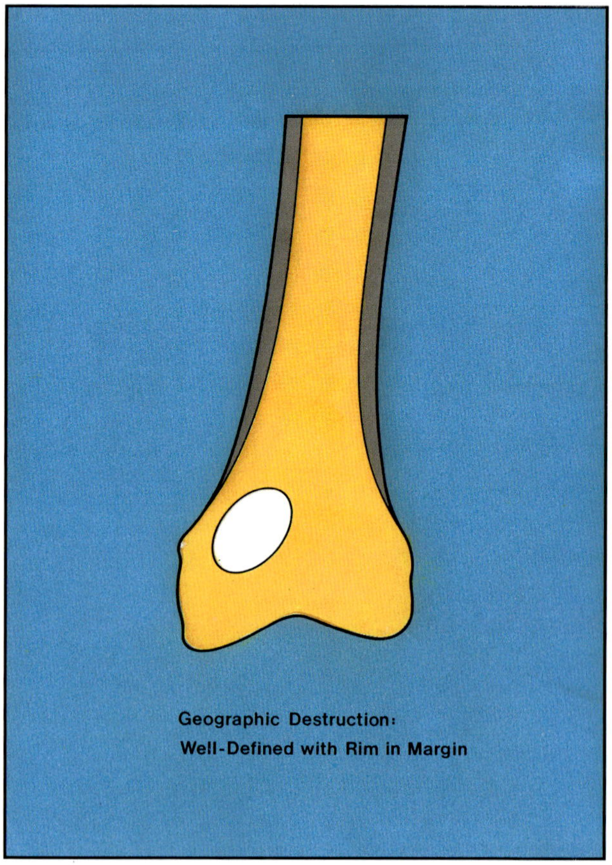

Figure 1-4

X-RAY MARGINS

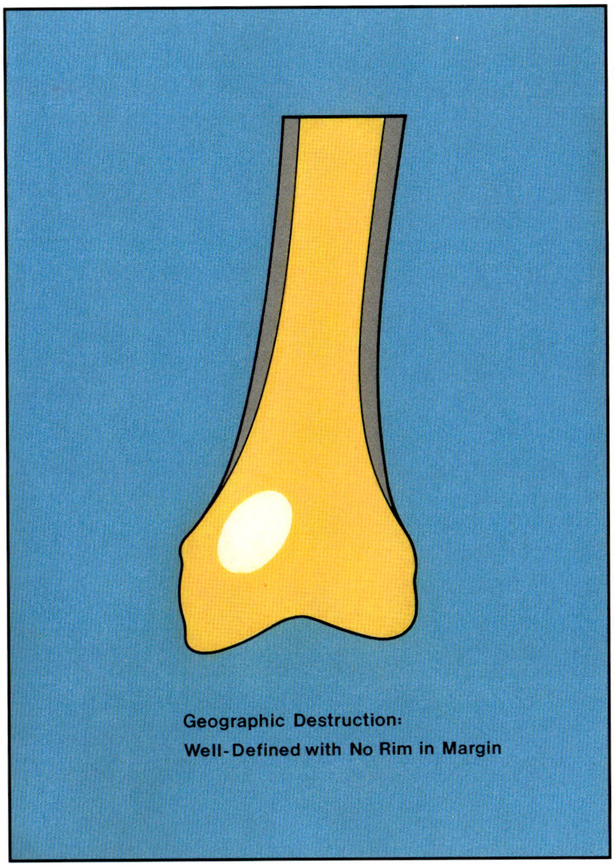

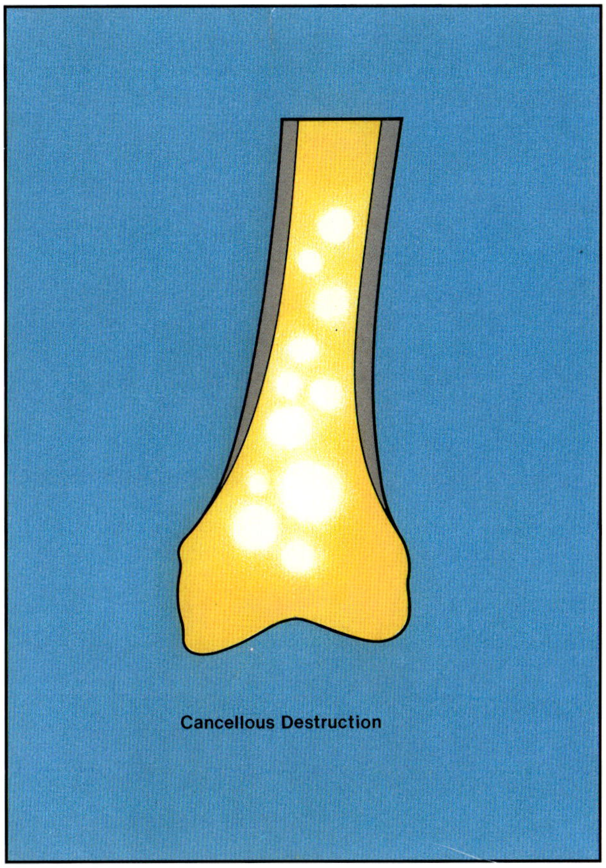

Figures 1-4, 1-5, 1-6. Sharply circumscribed. The lesion is clearly definable; one is able to draw a sharp pencil line about the confines of the destructive process (Figure 1-4). There may or may not be a reactive rim of bone about the lesion (Figure 1-5). There may be multiple lesions, all slow growing (enchondromas) (Figure 1-6).

sponse of the host bone to slow to rapid removal of the cortex of the affected bone. A rapid destructive pattern (permeative destruction) will result in a rapidly formed periosteal reaction, such as a Codman triangle, "hair on end," or "onion-peel". Conversely, if the process is slow growing, enough time remains for bone to reinforce the external margin, and thickening of the cortex or "buttress formation" results. Again, these characteristics do not imply a diagnosis; they only indicate the

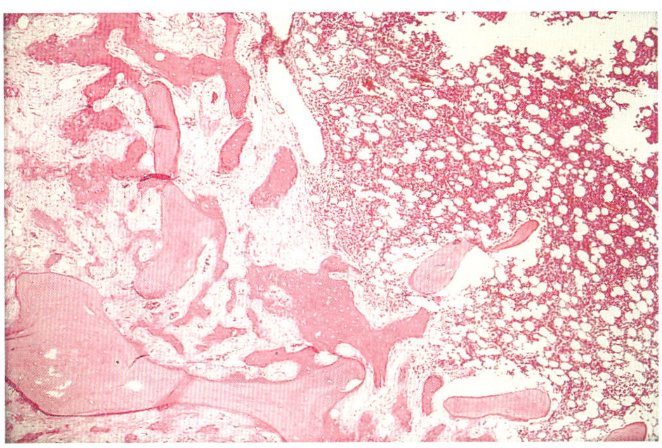

Figure 1-7. X-ray margins: moth-eaten. A mixture of residual trabecular bone and neoplastic new bone accompanied by mildly cellular fibrous connective tissue. Although there is no reactive rim of bone surrounding the margin, the process extends partially into the adjacent bony and hematopoietic marrow. Normal hematopoietic marrow is present, just beyond the infiltrating tumor. Radiographically this should be a moth-eaten margin.

X-RAY MARGINS

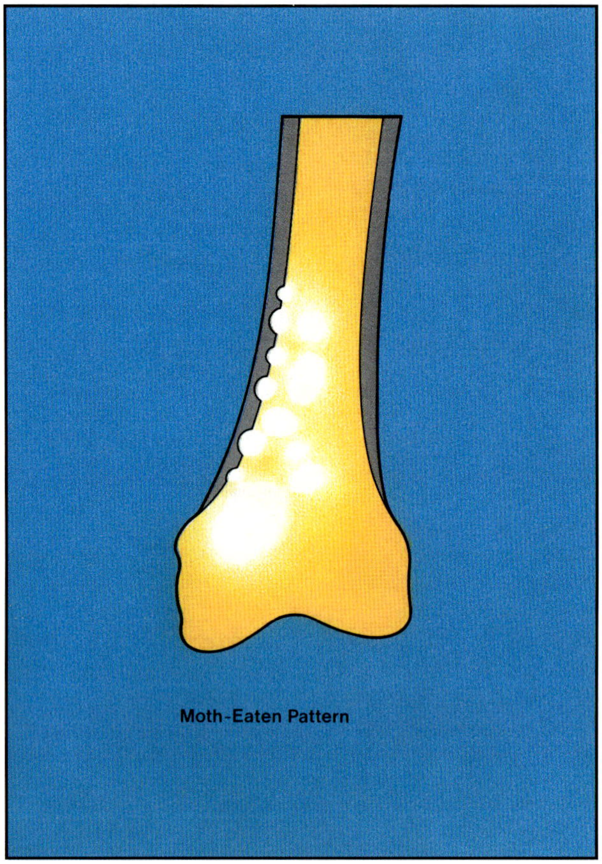

Figure 1-8. Moth-eaten margins exhibit indefinite margins which cannot be sharply defined. Small chunks seem to be taken out of the bone adjacent to the lesion, and this implies moderately aggressive growth pattern. The destructive pattern may be confined to the bone itself, or may involve the endosteal margin of the cortex, in which case one refers to endosteal scalloping. These moth-eaten destructive patterns indicate an aggressive pattern, consistent with a slow-growing malignant process.

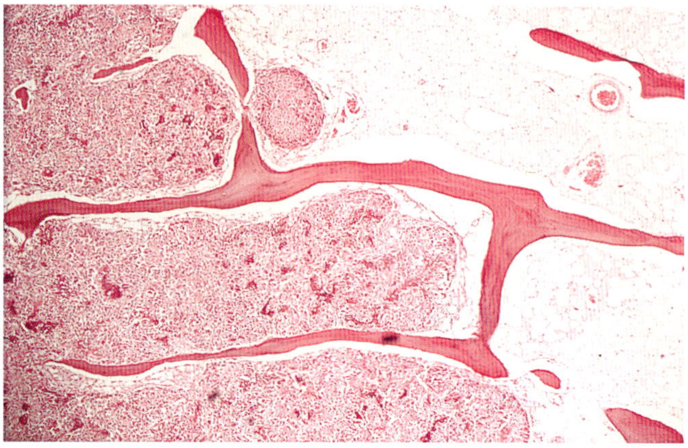

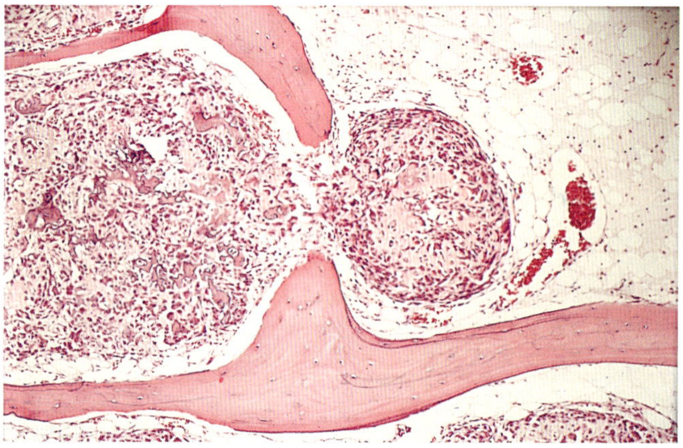

Figures 1-9, 1-10. A&B X-ray margin: permeative. The process infiltrates between trabeculae into adjacent marrow. Neoplastic osteoid production is easily identified. The trabeculae remain more or less intact without any effort to remodel and contain the tumor. The radiographs will therefore demonstrate the normal trabecular pattern with only minimal loss of bone, i.e., permeative destruction.

rapidity of the process that destroys bone. The radiologist equates rapidity with the likelihood of a malignant process, and slow growing changes in the bone with the likelihood of a benign process (Figures 1-13 to 1-19).

3. *Matrix production.* The presence or absence of identifiable matrix calcification produced by the neoplasm affords a clue as to whether one is dealing with an osteoid or cartilaginous neoplasm (Figures 1-20, 1-21).

Radiographic principles of analysis are obviously more complicated than stated above. To the novice, these sound imposing, but pathologists must not be overwhelmed and turn away from understanding basic principles of radiographic analysis and radiographic descriptive terminology. More important, there are histologic features that can predict these radiographic features. Thus if the lesion exhibits a permeative or moth-eaten pattern of destruction, the histologic picture at the edge of the lesion should show an invasive propensity with neoplastic or inflammatory tissue extending into the adjacent normal marrow (Figures 1-9, 1-10). If the lesion is sharply circumscribed on the radiograph, then there should be a very distinct margin of lesional tissue, with sharp separation from adjacent normal trabecular bone and marrow (Figure 1-3). If there is a rim of reactive bone visible on the biopsy, this should also be seen on the x-ray. An indistinct margin on the slide corresponds to moth-eaten margin on the radiograph

X-RAY MARGINS

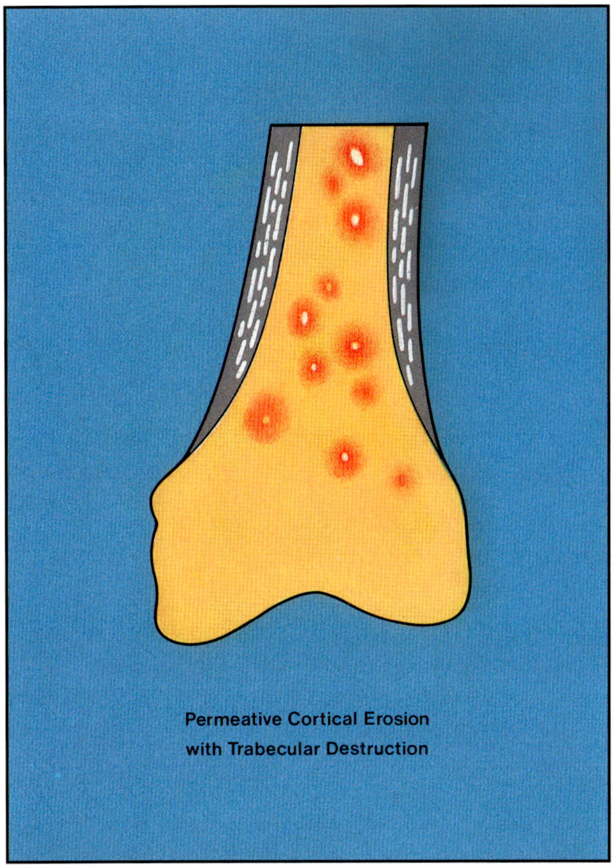

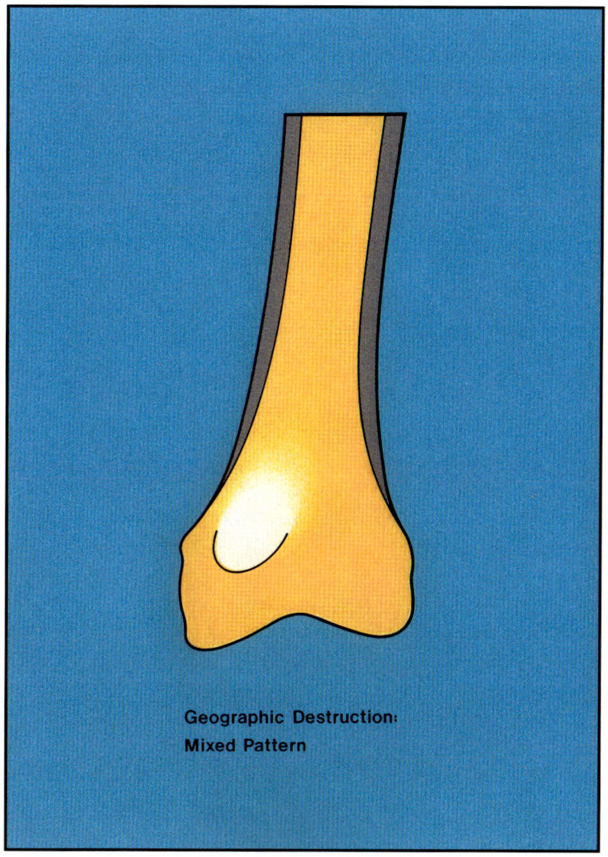

Figures 1-11, 1-12. Permeative destruction is rapid. It permeates through the trabecular bone, and establishes cutting cones throughout the cortex. A mixture of these pattern may well be present in any given lesion, implying different rates of growth at different sites.

(Figure 1-7). If calcification is present within the lesion, then there has to be some calcified tissue in the biopsy, and the presence of calcification in radiographs should automatically signal a search for the same calcified material in the biopsy material, such as the pathologist searches for calcification in a breast biopsy. In short, the pathologist should review the microscopic appearance of the lesion and be able to predict the radiograph.

There are distinct geographic areas where the tumor or anomaly has its characteristic home (Figures 1-22, 1-23). These reflect the field of the normal progenitor cell. Thus, chondroblastomas are always epiphyseal; the location reflects the site of chondroblast proliferation in the growing skeleton. Osteoclasts, from which giant cell tumors develop, are metaphyseal, and resorb calcified cartilage and primary trabeculae on the metaphyseal side of the growth plate before extending into the epiphysis. Giant cell tumors are therefore metaphyseal and epiphyseal. Fibrohistiocytic and osteoblastic tumors are usually metaphyseal. Round cell tumors are often diaphyseal, reflecting marrow origin. While these are generalizations, and not true in every case, it is difficult if not impossible to visualize a metaphyseal or diaphyseal chondroblastoma. With extremely rare exceptions,[14,15] giant cell tumor of bone is associated with a growth plate. If a diaphyseal giant cell tumor is identified, there is a strong likelihood that one is dealing with a brown tumor of hyperparathyroidism rather than a bona fide giant cell tumor of bone. Fibrous dysplasia or unicameral bone cyst are anomalies arising at the growth plate, and are always a centrally located lesion once they have progressed beyond the first few weeks; the lesion should involve the entire width of the bone. It is uncommon if not impossible to have eccentrically located unicameral bone cyst or fibrous dysplasia; one would have to question the appropriateness of that diagnosis. The typical

X-RAY MARGINS

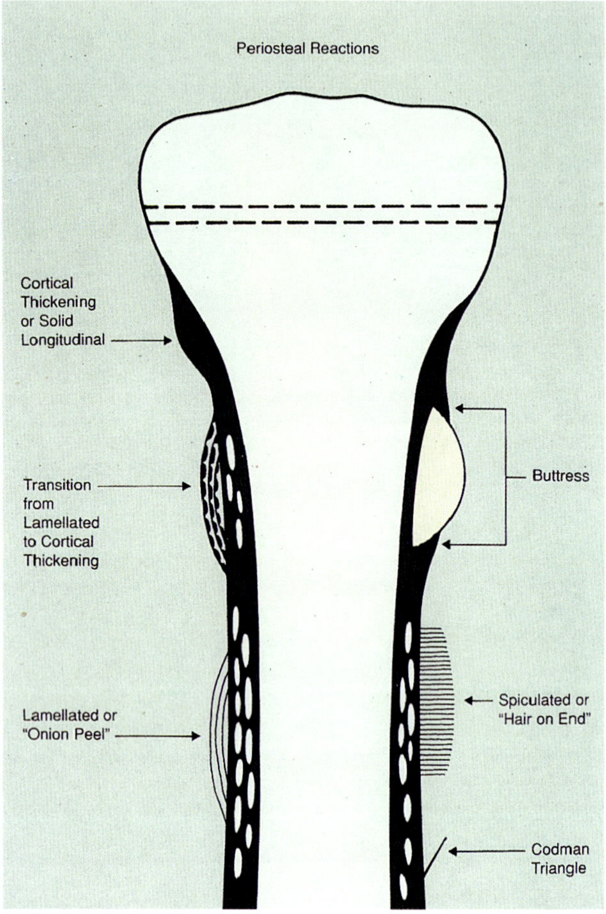

Figure 1-13. Composite diagram of periosteal reactions.

location and characteristics for all of these neoplastic and anomalous processes are identified in Figures 1-22 and 1-23, and require correlation with the biopsy diagnosis.

The ultimate diagnosis that is given to any lesion of bone depends exclusively upon its histologic appearance at the time of biopsy. The tissue diagnosis is the ultimate responsibility of a pathologist. All other factors are correlative studies; however, they cannot be ignored, therefore histologic diagnosis that does not fit into a known pattern of radiographic appearance is suspect. The pathologist must be very careful to eliminate all other possibilities before rendering a firm diagnosis in the case of an atypical presentation. Clinical data is similar. While the age and sex of the patient and location of the process within the bone follow predictable epidemiologic data, statistical data is not, and should not be used to establish a diagnosis. It is simply the "Las Vegas line" on a given lesion; one should not ignore the odds maker, but long shots do exist. There are occasional 40-year-old patients with diaphyseal osteosarcoma (Figures 1-24, 1-25).

Staging

Tumors arising in bone often have a characteristic or predictable biologic behavior and pattern of growth. These patterns form the basis of a staging system and current treatment strategies. These principles and their relationship to management were formulated by Enneking in 1980 and updated by him in 1986.[16,17]

Biology and Growth

On the basis of biologic considerations and natural history, Enneking classified bone tumors into five categories, each of which share certain clinical characteristics, radiographic patterns, and similar surgical therapeutic procedures.

a. *Benign/Latent:* Lesions that grow slowly during normal growth of the person and then stop with a tendency to heal spontaneously. These lesions almost never become malignant, and if treated by simple curettage, heal rapidly. Surgery is not indicated unless they become symptomatic.

b. *Benign/Active:* Lesions that have a natural history of progressive growth. Simple curettage of this lesion leaves a rim of reactive bone with some tumor. Curettage has a high recurrence rate. Wide excision through normal bone results in local control in approximately 95% of the cases.

c. *Benign/Aggressive:* Lesions that are locally aggressive but do not metastasize. Pathologically there is tumor extension through the capsule into the reactive zone. Local control can be obtained only by removing the lesion with a margin of normal bone beyond the reactive zone.

d. *Malignant/Low Grade:* Lesions that have a low potential to metastasize. Histologically, there is no true capsule but a pseudocapsule. Tumor nodules exist within the reactive zone, but rarely beyond. Local control can be accomplished only by removal of all tumor and reactive tissue with a margin of normal bone. These lesions can be treated effectively by surgery alone; systemic chemotherapy is often not required.

e. *Malignant/High Grade:* Lesions have a natural history of rapid growth and early metastasis. Characteristically, tumor nodules are found within and beyond the reactive zone and at some distance in the normal tissue (i.e., satellite lesions and skip metastases). Surgery is

PERIOSTEAL REACTIONS

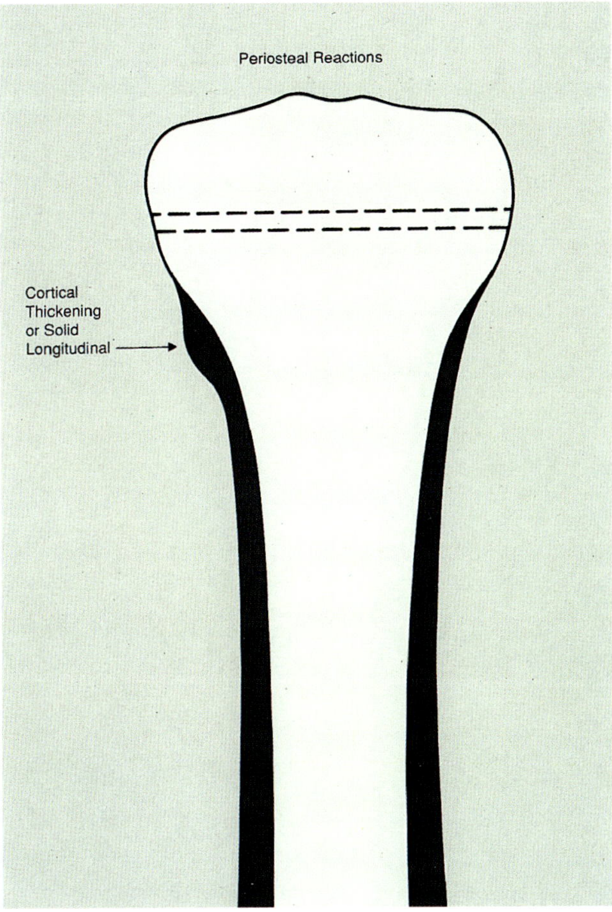

Figure 1-14. Cortical thickening. Periosteal reactions vary with the speed of the destructive pattern. Thus the slow process, i.e., benign, will cause a slow expansion of cortex and reinforcement of the cortical margin. The slow expansion leads to additional bone formation, thickening the cortex in a solid longitudinal pattern. An example of this cortical thickening is the "saber-shin" of syphilis.

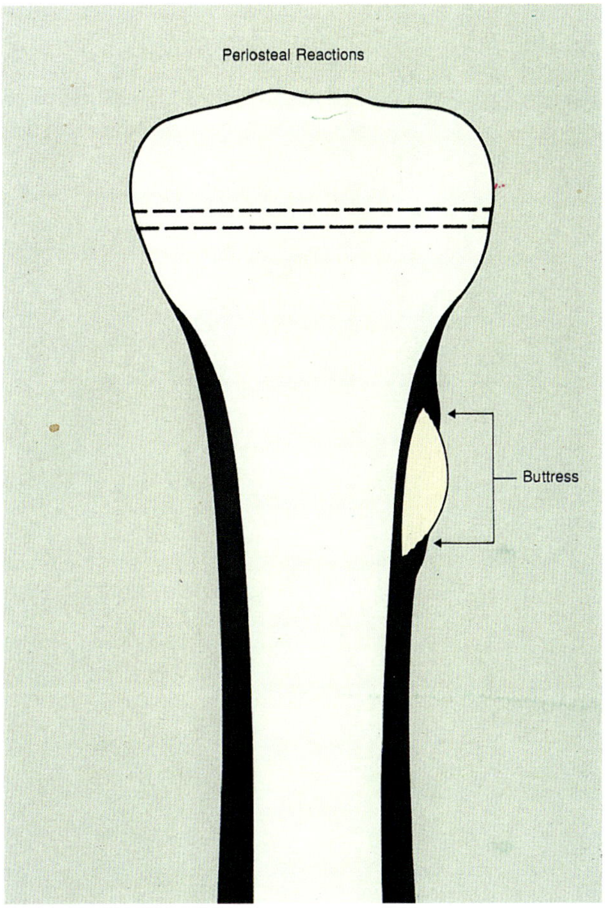

Figure 1-15. Buttress formation. Of equally slow nature is the so-called buttress formation. The lesion itself may be present for some time, localized on the periosteal surface. On either side of this surface lesion there is thickening of bone, solidifying over many months.

necessary for local control, and systemic therapy is warranted to treat metastases.

Metastasis
Unlike carcinomas, sarcomas of bone disseminate almost exclusively through the blood. There are only rare cases of spread to the regional lymph nodes. Hematogenous spread is manifested by pulmonary involvement in its early stages and secondarily by bony involvement. Occasionally, bone metastasis is the first sign of dissemination.

Skip Metastasis
A skip metastasis is a tumor nodule that is located within the same bone as the main tumor, but is not in continuity with it. Skip lesions are seen most often with high grade lesions. A skip lesion develops by embolization of tumor cells within the marrow sinusoids, and they are in effect, local micrometastases that have not passed through the systemic circulation.

Local Recurrence
Local recurrence is due to incomplete removal and subsequent regrowth of either a benign or malignant lesion. Adequacy of surgical removal is the main determinant of local control. The aggressiveness of the lesion and

PERIOSTEAL REACTIONS

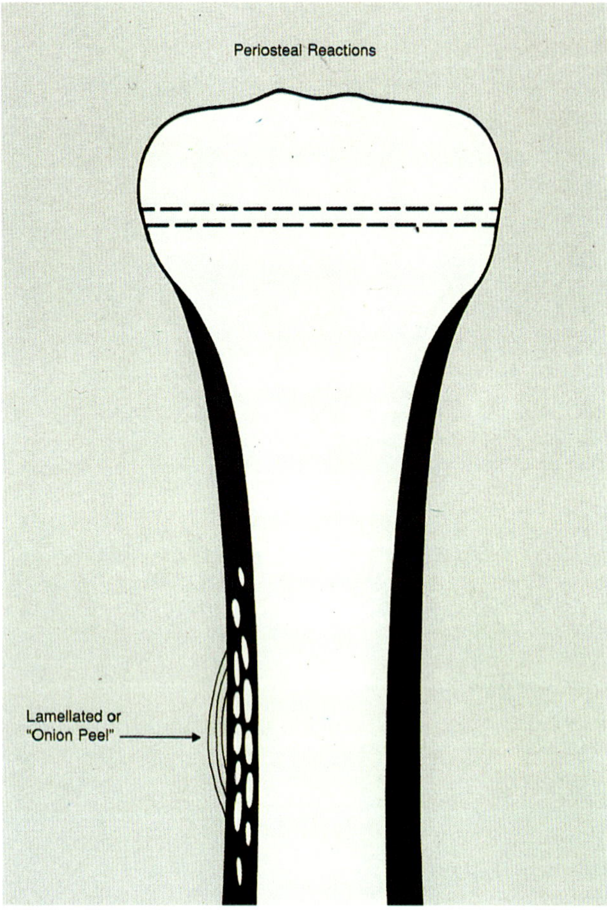

Figure 1-16

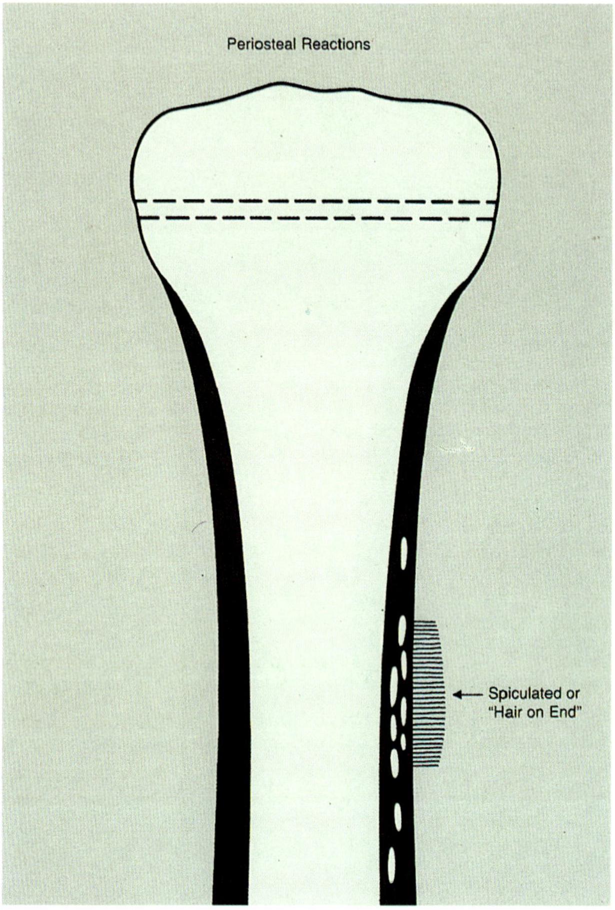

Figure 1-17

Figure 1-16, 1-17, 1-18, 1-19. The more rapidly growing processes may develop several types of periosteal reactions. Any periosteal reaction is a response to loss of cortical bone. Cortical bone may be destroyed or remodeled by many processes; the attempt to repair is preceded by the necessity to remove existing bone, which often results in the formation of the "cutting cone." Cutting cones represent rapid destruction and remodeling of the cortex, and may be seen in fracture, stress fracture, or osteomyelitis, but also in any of the neoplastic processes. The reinforcement of the weakened cortex is accomplished by sending out streamers of new bone, which ultimately fill in and become solid. Thus in the initial phase of rapid destruction of bone, the periosteum may react by forming either "onion-peel" (Figure 1-16) or streamers of bone ("hair-on-end") (Figure 1-17) or a partial streamer, the Codman triangle (Figure 1-18). All of these manifestations indicate rapid destruction of the underlying cortex, as seen in Ewing's sarcoma, osteosarcoma, or in an inflammatory process. If the destructive process in the bone is arrested, the periosteal reaction will solidify and become a thickened cortex indicating its arrested and self-limited nature (Figure 1-19). If the process continues to destroy the cortical bone, successive onion peels or additional hair-on-end (sunburst) periosteal reactions will continue to form. The extent of the periosteal reaction is simply an indication of the speed with which the underlying bone is being destroyed. No diagnosis can be attached to the presence or absence of a sunburst, onion-peel, or Codman triangle per se.

PERIOSTEAL REACTIONS

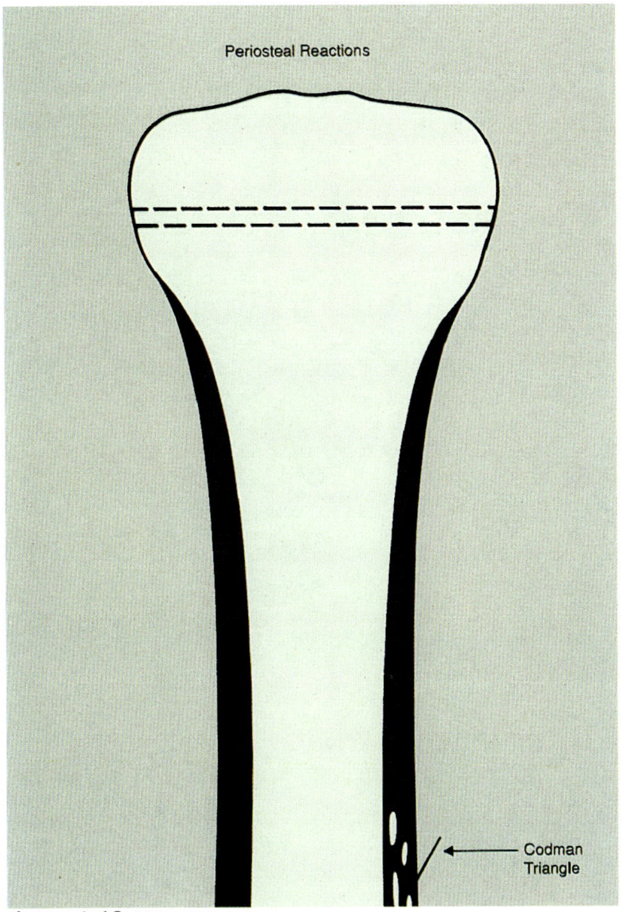

Figure 1-18

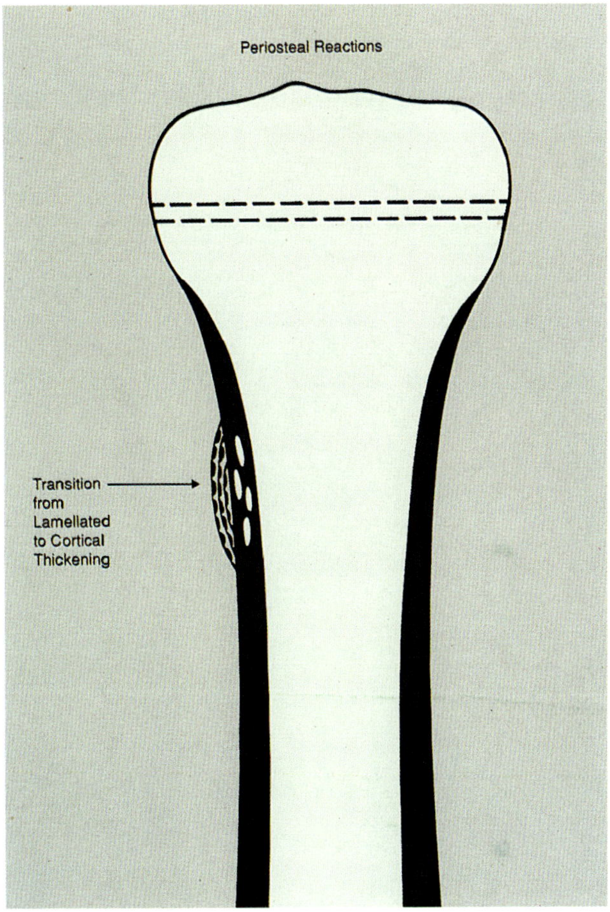

Figure 1-19

thereby its clinical stage determines which surgical procedure is required for local control.

Surgical Staging System (Enneking)

In 1980, the Musculoskeletal Tumor Society adopted a Surgical Staging System (SSS) for bone and soft tissue sarcomas. This SSS described by Enneking and coworkers[16,17] is based upon the GTM classification: grade (G), location (T), and metastases (M).

Surgical Grade (G): In malignant tumors, G represents the histologic grade of a lesion and other clinical data used to make a surgical determination of low grade (GI) or high grade (GII).

In this grading system the grade assigned to the sarcoma is not based on histologic criteria alone; the generally accepted biologic behavior of the entity contributes to the grade. Thus, Ewing's sarcoma is always grade II regardless of its histology. Intramedullary osteosarcoma is grade II; typical parosteal osteosarcoma is grade I.

Benign tumors are graded on the basis of activity rather than histology. Grade 1 benign tumors, such as nonossifying fibroma, are dormant or latent intracompartmental lesions with little or no chance of expansion. Grade 2 benign lesions include unicameral bone cysts. These are intracompartmental lesions but they have a tendency to slowly but steadily increase in size. Grade 3 benign lesions are aggressive, tend to extend beyond a single anatomical compartment, and frequently recur. Occasionally, cells from Grade 3 lesions are transported to the lungs (implants) as may be seen with some examples of giant cell tumors and chondroblastomas.

Surgical Site (T): T represents anatomical site, either intracompartmental (T1) or extracompartmental (T2). Compartment is defined as an anatomic structure or space bound by natural barriers of tumor extension (Table 1-1).

CALCIFICATION PATTERNS

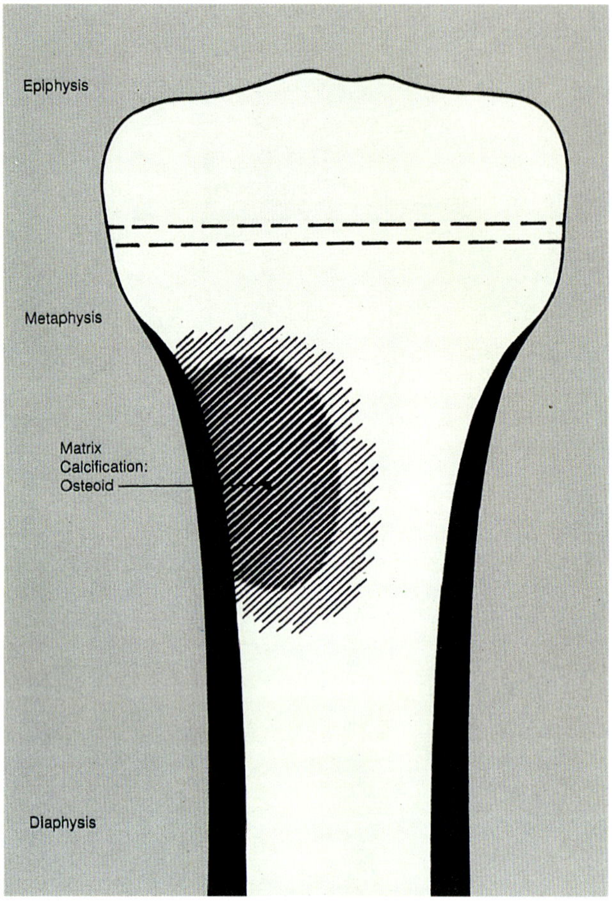

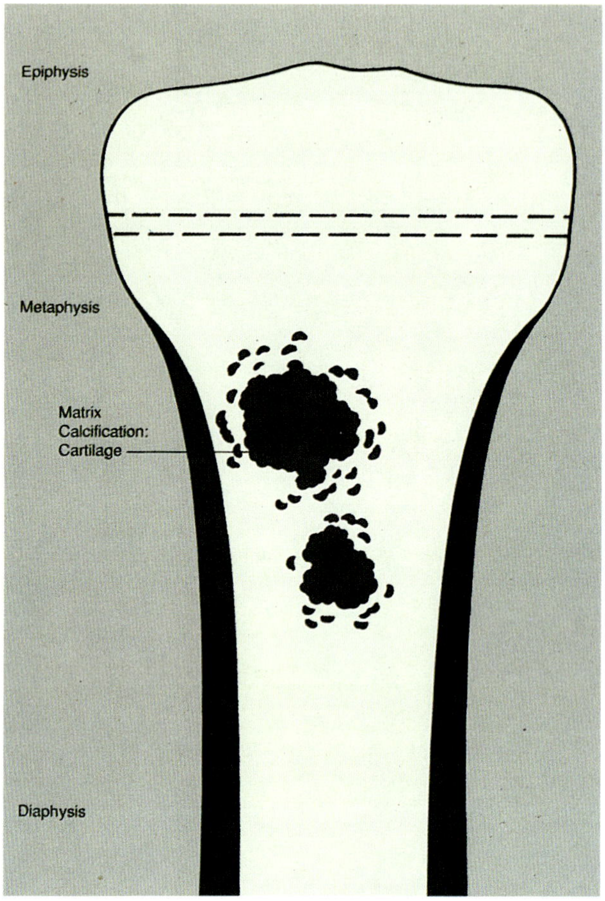

Figures 1-20, 1-21. The calcification of a neoplastic process is an indication of its tissue of origin. Thus osteosarcomas or osteoblastic lesions of any kind will tend to form streamers of bone, with a linear calcification process (Figure 1-20). Cartilage will calcify in a flocculent pattern, very much like plaster of Paris sticking against the wall (Figure 1-21).

Metastasis (M): Regional or distant, lymph node, pulmonary or other.

The staging system for malignant lesions may be summarized as follows:

Stage IA (G1, T1, M0): Low grade, intracompartmental lesion without metastasis.

Stage IB (G1, T2, M0): Low grade, extracompartmental lesion without metastasis.

Stage IIA (G2, T1, M0): High grade, intracompartmental lesion without metastasis.

Stage IIB (G2, T2, M0): High grade, extracompartmental lesion without metastasis.

Stage IIIA (G1 or G2, T1, M1): Intracompartmental lesions, any grade, with metastasis.

Stage IIIB (G1 or G2, T2, M1): Extracompartmental lesions, any grade, with metastasis.

Most osteosarcomas are stage IIB when they first present; they are high grade lesions (G2) by virtue of their known biologic behavior. If they extend outside the bone they are extracompartmental (T2). If there are no distant metastases (M0), the lesion is stage IIB. If there are metastases, the same tumor is stage IIIB.

Benign Tumors
Grade

1. Latent
   a. Intracompartmental
   b. Extracompartmental

CALCIFICATION PATTERNS

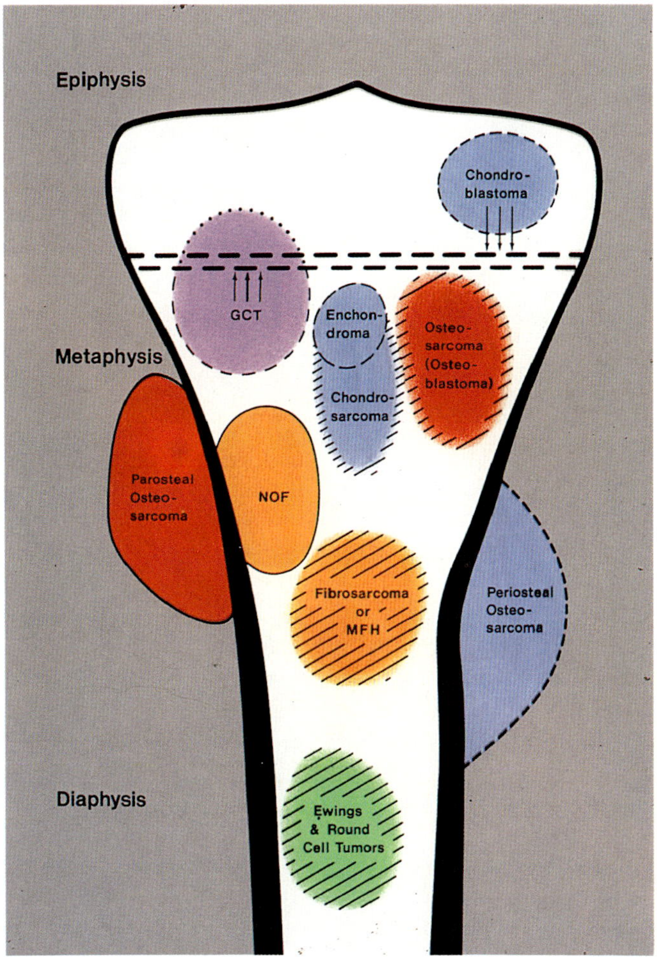

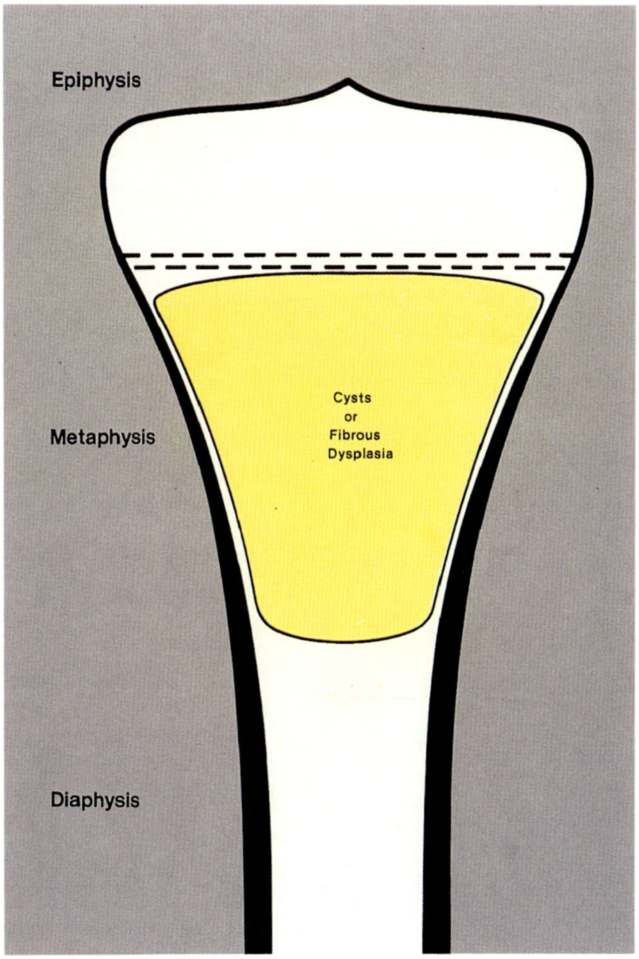

Figure 1-22, 1-23. Classical locations of osseous neoplasms, reflecting the site of the normal cellular activity.

2. Active
   a. Intracompartmental
   b. Extracompartmental
3. Aggressive
   a. Intracompartmental
   b. Extracompartmental

Management

Definitive diagnosis determines the sequence and nature of the therapeutic steps. Certain lesions are treated with adjuvant or neoadjuvant chemotherapy. Other lesions require radiation therapy with chemotherapy, and surgery plays only a secondary role. Conversely, some lesions are not amenable to any pre- or postoperative chemotherapy, and require a purely surgical approach. Infectious lesions require relief of pressure (accomplished by open biopsy) and appropriate therapy with anti-inflammatory agents.

Every biopsy requires a culture, and every culture requires a biopsy. It is often difficult to differentiate between lymphoma, Ewing's sarcoma, and osteomyelitis; not only do the lesions present similar radiographic appearance, but the "fish-flesh" appearance of Ewing's sarcoma can be mistaken for pus from an osteomyelitis and vice versa. Thus the pathologist should remind the surgeon that any biopsy requires a culture, and conversely, if bone is entered for the purpose of relieving intraosseous pressure in a suspected osteomyelitis, a biopsy should be taken as well.

CALCIFICATION PATTERNS

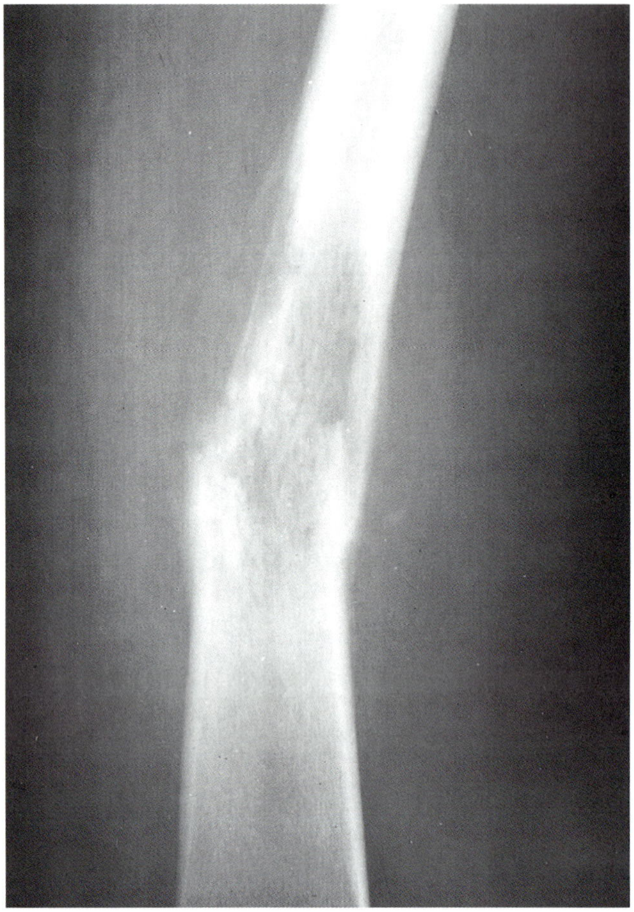

Figure 1-24. Thirty-six-year-old female patient complaining of pain in knee. Fracture during physiotherapy. Permeative lytic destruction of diaphyseal portion of femur, Codman triangle, and pathologic fracture.

Surgical Management of Skeletal Tumors

Surgical options include curettage, resection, or amputation as the traditional methods of tumor management. More recently, limb-sparing techniques have been developed.[5,18,19] Enneking and coworkers have formulated a scheme of classification of surgical procedures.[16,17] This classification permits meaningful comparison of various operative procedures and serves as the basis of a common language.

1. *Intralesional (Intracapsular):* An intralesional procedure passes through the pseudocapsule of the neoplasm and directly into the lesion. Macroscopic tumor remains and the entire operative field is potentially contaminated. Curettage is an example of intralesional procedure.

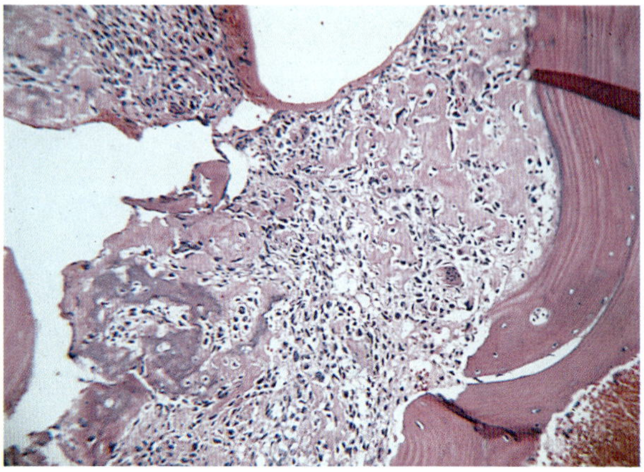

Figure 1-25. Osteosarcoma: histologic examination of the diaphyseal pathologic fracture in this patient, exhibiting an osteosarcoma. This patient was not aware of the Las Vegas odds. Diagnosis depends on histologic analysis of the lesion!

2. *Marginal:* A marginal procedure is one in which the entire lesion is removed in one piece. The plane of dissection passes through the pseudocapsule or reactive zone around the lesion. When performed for a sarcoma, a marginal procedure has a high likelihood of residual microscopic disease leading to recurrence.

TABLE 1-1. Staging of Musculoskeletal Sarcomas

Surgical Sites (T)	
Intracompartmental (T1)	*Extracompartmental (T2)*
Intraosseous	Soft-tissue extension
Intra-articular	Soft-tissue extension
Superficial to deep fascia	Deep fascial extension
Paraosseous	Intraosseous or extrafascial
Intrafascial compartments	Extrafascial planes or spaces
Ray of hand or foot	Mid and hind foot
Posterior calf	Popliteal space
Anterolateral leg	Groin-femoral triangle
Medial thigh	Intrapelvic
Posterior thigh	Mid-hand
Buttocks	Antecubital fossae
Volar forearm	Axilla
Dorsal forearm	Periclavicular
Anterior arm	Paraspinal
Posterior arm	Head and neck
Periscapular	

Reproduced from ref. 13, p. 17.

CALCIFICATION PATTERNS

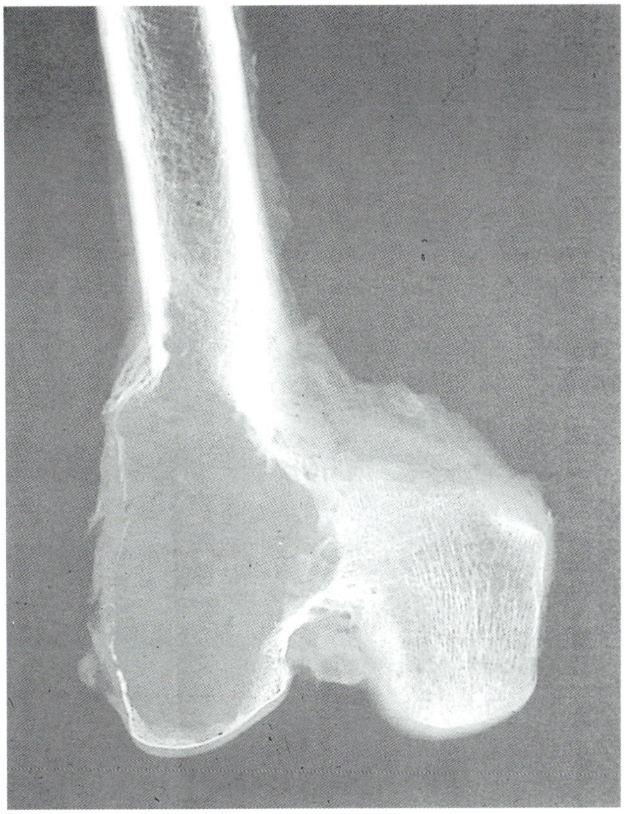

Figure 1-26. Specimen x-ray of postoperative curetted giant cell tumor of femoral condyle.

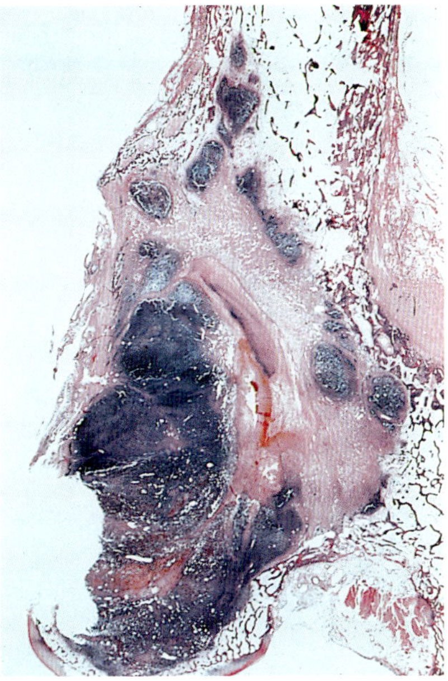

Figure 1-27. Macrospecimen of Figure 1-26. Residual tumor has filled the previously curetted cavity, and additional nodules of tumor are present beyond the original curettement cavity.

3. *Wide (Intracompartmental):* A wide excision includes the entire tumor, the reactive zone, and a cuff of normal tissue. The entire compartment is not removed. This is commonly referred to as en bloc resection.
4. *Radical (Extracompartmental):* The entire tumor and structures of origin of the lesion are removed. The plane of dissection is beyond the limiting fascial or bony borders.

The local anatomy determines how a specific margin should be obtained. Therefore the aim of preoperative staging is to assess local tumor extent and important local anatomy to permit determination of how a desired margin is to be achieved, and thus determine the feasibility of one surgical procedure over another.

Resection
The pathologist will be requested to answer the following:

In the case of resection, is the lesion completely excised? How effective is preoperative chemotherapy?

The pathologist has no difficulty in determining whether a lesion of the breast or colon is completely excised. The surgeon usually presents tissue and asks for frozen section of the margin. The same standard of practice should prevail in resected bone lesions. In many instances the orthopaedic surgeon will perform an intralesional excision, i.e., curettage, and attempt to sterilize the margins of the curettement through the use of heat, cryosurgery, phenol, or other agents which penetrate through the adjacent tissue and effectively eliminate all viable cellular material. Postoperative films can usually determine whether these margins are indeed curetted, and the persistence of a sharp margin unchanged from the preoperative study would tend to suggest that the lesion was not completely curetted. The pathologist can ask the surgeon to perform the curettage, then go back and provide additional curetted material from the margin of the cavity which can be processed separately and reviewed for remaining neoplastic material. While the intralesional excision is never complete cancer surgery, an opinion can be made as to whether the lesion is likely to recur. Local recurrence is, unfortunately, nothing other than incomplete excision (Figures 1-26, 1-27).

POST-CHEMOTHERAPY EVALUATION

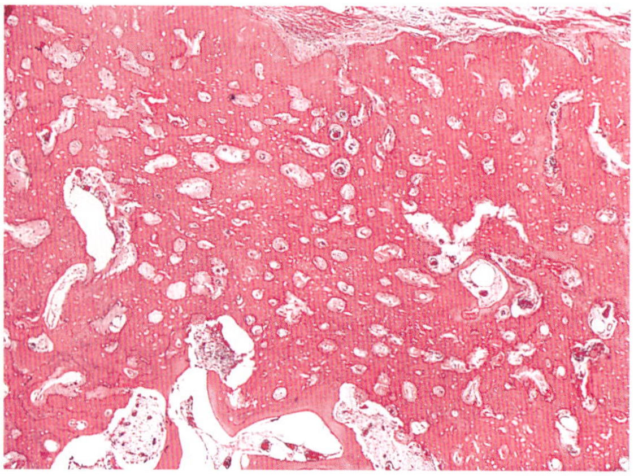

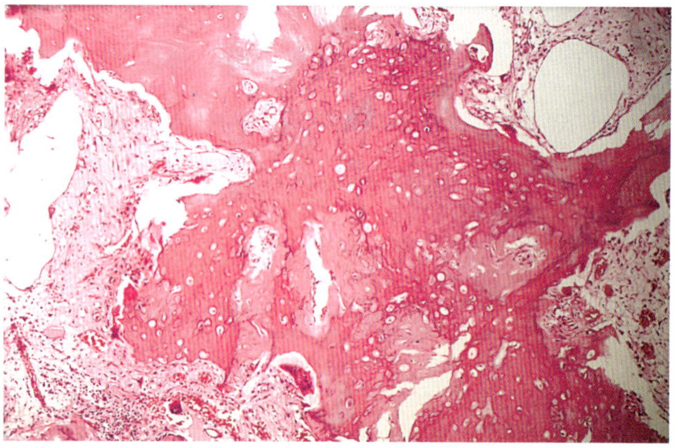

Figures 1-28, 1-29. Osteosarcoma after therapy with chemotherapy. While the osteoid may remain, all cellular elements have disappeared leaving behind empty lacunae ("turtle shells"). At least 95% of the resected specimen should show this pattern for therapy to be considered successful.

Wide excision is an attempt to resect the neoplasm and the rim of reactive tissue bordering the lesion, and to extend completely into adjacent normal tissue. These margins should be inked, and always examined for adequacy of excision. Of particular interest is the margin of a segmental resection of bone. The marrow cavity is often the site of more extensive spread, not necessarily clearly definable on the radiograph, CAT scan, or MRI study. Thus if a limb salvage procedure resects portions of the femoral head and neck, the marrow cavity at the distal end of such a resection should always be submitted for frozen section at the time of the procedure. It would be futile to amputate or partially resect major portions of bone only to have local recurrence at the site of the transected bone.

It is important to understand the effect that chemotherapy will have on neoplastic processes. The effect of neoadjuvant (preoperative) chemotherapy has to be assessed, in order to allow the oncologist to decide whether to modify dosage, discontinue, or require additional agents when administering adjuvant therapy. This is accomplished by histologically assessing the viability of the residual tumor following neoadjuvant therapy. In the hands of centers with extensive experience in neoadjuvant chemotherapy, 95% death of tumor cell is considered the minimal threshold for considering a lesion successfully treated.[7,12,20–26] Anything less requires either a change in chemotherapy, additional chemotherapy, or other modes of treatment. The pathologist must therefore take a resected specimen, map it out, and assess the total percentage of necrotic cells, field by field, until the entire lesion has been quantitatively examined (Figures 1-28, 1-29).

In the field of orthopaedic tumor surgery the role of the pathologist has greatly expanded with the advent of combined adjuvant and neoadjuvant therapy, limb salvage procedures, and the role of radiation therapy. One must welcome the really significant improvement in survival and the preservation of extremities. The future will present challenges in earlier evaluation of response to chemotherapy. The pathologist must live up to the new responsibilities and future challenges.[2,5,20,21,27–30]

REFERENCES

1. Matthews JG: Principles of biopsy and resection of musculoskeletal tumors. In Chapman MW (ed): *Operative Orthopaedics,* ed 2. Philadelphia, Lippincott, 1993, pp 2483–2494.
2. Simon MA, Finn HA: Diagnostic strategy for bone and soft-tissue. *J Bone Joint Surg* 75A(4):622–631, 1993.
3. Resnick D, Niwayama G: *Diagnosis of Bone and Joint Disorders.* ed 2. Philadelphia, WB Saunders, 1988, p 2022.
4. Carter SR, Grimer RJ, Sneath RS: A review of 13-years experience of osteosarcoma. *Clin Orthop Relat Res* 270: 45–51, 1991.
5. Simon MA: Limb salvage for osteosarcoma in the 1980s. *Clin Orthop Relat Res* 270:264–270, 1991.
6. Veth RP: IIB osteosarcoma. Current management, local control, and survival statistics—The Netherlands. *Clin Orthop Relat Res* 270:67–71, 1991.
7. Winkler K, Bieling P, Bielack S, et al: Local control and survival from the Cooperative Osteosarcoma Study Group studies of the German Society of Pediatric Oncology and

the Vienna Bone Tumor Registry. *Clin Orthop Relat Res* 270:79–86, 1991.

8. Simon MA, Biermann JS: Biopsy of bone and soft tissue. *J Bone Joint Surg* 75A(4):616–621, 1993.
9. Layfield LJ, Armstrong K, Zaleski S, et al: Diagnostic accuracy and clinical utility of fine-needle aspiration cytology in the diagnosis of clinically primary bone lesions. *Diagn Cytopath* 9(2):168–173, 1993.
10. Davies NM, Livesley PJ, Cannon SR: Recurrence of an osteosarcoma in a needle biopsy track. *J Bone Joint Surg Br* 75(6):977–978, 1993.
11. Madewell JE, Ragsdale BD, Sweet DE: Radiologic and pathologic analysis of solitary bone lesions. Part I: Internal margins. *Radiol Clin North Amer* 19:715–747, 1981.
12. Ragsdale BD, Madewell JE, Sweet DE: Radiologic and pathology analysis of solitary bone lesions. Part II: Periosteal reactions. *Radiol Clin North Amer* 19:749–783, 1981.
13. Sweet DE, Madewell JE, Ragsdale BD: Radiologic and pathologic analysis of solitary bone lesions. Part III: Matrix patterns. *Radiol Clin North Amer* 19:785–814, 1981.
14. Bertoni F, Unni KK, Beabout JW, et al: Giant cell tumor of the skull. *Cancer* 70(5):1124–1132, 1992.
15. Fain JS, Unni KK, Beabout JW, et al: Non-epiphyseal giant cell tumor of the long bones. Clinical, radiologic, and pathologic study. *Cancer* 71(11):3514–3519, 1993.
16. Enneking WF: A system of staging musculoskeletal neoplasms. *Clin Orthop* 204:6–24, 1986.
17. Enneking WF, Spanier SS, Goodman MA: A system for the surgical staging of musculoskeletal sarcoma. *Clin Orthop* 153:106–120, 1980.
18. Eilber FR, Mirra JJ, Grant TT, et al: Is amputation necessary for sarcomas? A seven-year study with limb salvage. *Ann Surg* 192:431, 1980.
19. Simon MA, Aschliman MA, Thomas N, et al: Limb-salvage treatment versus amputation for osteosarcoma of the distal end of the femur. *J Bone Joint Surg* 68A:1331–1337, 1986.
20. Edeline V, Frouin F, Bazin JP, et al: Factor analysis as a means of determining response to chemotherapy in patients with osteogenic sarcoma. *Eur J Nucl Med* 20(12): 1175–1185, 1993.
21. Goorin AM, Andersen JW: Experience with multiagent chemotherapy for osteosarcoma. Improved outcome. *Clin Orthop Relat Res* 270:22–28, 1991.
22. Huvos AG, Rosen G, Marcove RC: Primary osteogenic sarcoma. Pathologic aspects in 20 patients after treatment with chemotherapy, en bloc resection, and prosthetic bone replacement. *Arch Pathol Lab Med* 101:14–18, 1977.
23. Link MP, Goorin AM, Miser AW, et al: The effect of adjuvant chemotherapy on relapse-free survival in patients with osteosarcoma of the extremity. *NEJM* 314:1600–1606, 1986.
24. Picci P, Bacci G, Campanacci M, et al: Histologic evaluation of necrosis in osteosarcoma induced by chemotherapy: regional mapping of viable and nonviable tumor. *Cancer* 56:1515, 1985.
25. Rosen G, Marcove RC, Caparros B, et al: Primary osteogenic sarcoma. The rationale for preoperative chemotherapy and delayed surgery. *Cancer* 43:2163–2177, 1979.
26. Rosen G, Loren GJ, Brien EW, et al: Serial thallium-201 scintigraphy in osteosarcoma. Correlation with tumor necrosis after preoperative chemotherapy. *Clin Orthop Relat Res* 293:302–306, 1993.
27. Bacci G, Picci P, Ferrari S, et al: Primary chemotherapy and delayed surgery for non-metastatic osteosarcoma of the extremities. Results in 164 patients preoperatively treated with high doses of methotrexate followed by cisplatin and doxorubicin. *Cancer* 72(11):3227–3238, 1993.
28. Eilber FR, Rosen G: Adjuvant chemotherapy for osteosarcoma. *Semin Oncol* 16(4):312–322, 1989.
29. Meyer WH: Recent developments in genetic mechanisms, assessment, and treatment of osteosarcomas. *Curr Opin Oncol* 3(4):689–693, 1991.
30. Meyer WH, Malawer MM: Osteosarcoma. Clinical features and evolving surgical and chemotherapeutic strategies. *Pediatr Clin North Amer* 38(2):317–348, 1991.

2

Benign Reactive Processes Mimicking Neoplasia

FRACTURE CALLUS

The initial period in the histology of fracture healing is characterized by resorption of the fracture fragments. Osteoclasts are admixed with residual mature bone fragments and granulation tissue. There is usually extensive hemorrhage.

As the fracture begins to heal, the initial resorptive phase is replaced by early procallus formation. This tissue is difficult to differentiate from neoplastic elements. It is characterized by spindled, markedly pleomorphic cellular elements, often exhibiting primitive osteoid formation. One of the clues that one is dealing with fracture callus rather than neoplasm is the incorporation of striated muscle fibers into the reparative process. A neoplasm tends to abut against striated muscle or other soft tissue elements, while in the process of fracture healing, muscle is incorporated into the primitive callus. In some instances the transformation from muscle to primitive cellular granulation tissue is identifiable histologically (Figures 2-1 to 2-4).

As the fracture callus matures the differentiation into osteoid becomes more apparent. One is able to discern osteocytes encasing themselves in osteocytic lacunae, or a seam of osteoblasts lining up along the side of a trabecula of bone. This is in sharp contrast to fibroblastic differentiation, in which the nucleus is located in the center of the fiber.

As the callus matures further, a phase of bone formation ensues, in which there is additional maturation of the osteoid with the formation of actual bone, as well as a loss of the undifferentiated cellular elements adjacent to the bone. *There must be consistent maturation of both the matrix-forming tissue and the adjacent connective tissue, and they must be in phase.* Thus when there is immature bone there may be cellular immature connective tissue adjacent to the bony trabeculae. On the other hand, if there is mature bone, the connective tissue adjacent to the bone should also be more mature, i.e., less cellular, with less pleomorphism, and formation of dilated vascular spaces. Discrepancy in the maturation process indicates a neoplastic rather than a reactive process. If the bone formation appears mature, moderately cellular, but without significant pleomorphism or mitotic activity, and there is solid, spindled, cellular tissue adjacent to the trabeculae, one is probably dealing with something other than reactive bone.

Bone formation is enhanced by low oxygen content, and the blood flow that is associated wtih fracture callus at this stage is sinusoidal, low turnover, low oxygen tension. The maturing fracture callus exhibits numerous sinusoidal spaces between the bony elements.

The formation of chondro-osseous bone is a uniform feature of all fracture callus. The amount of cartilage that is formed in any fracture depends upon the vascularization of the fracture field, as well as the degree of motion within the fracture itself. Cartilage is a nonvascular tissue; it receives all its nutrition by diffusion, and it is therefore capable of dividing and reproducing without a direct capillary blood supply. Motion within the frac-

EARLY FRACTURE CALLUS VERSUS OSTEOSARCOMA, MIXED PATTERN

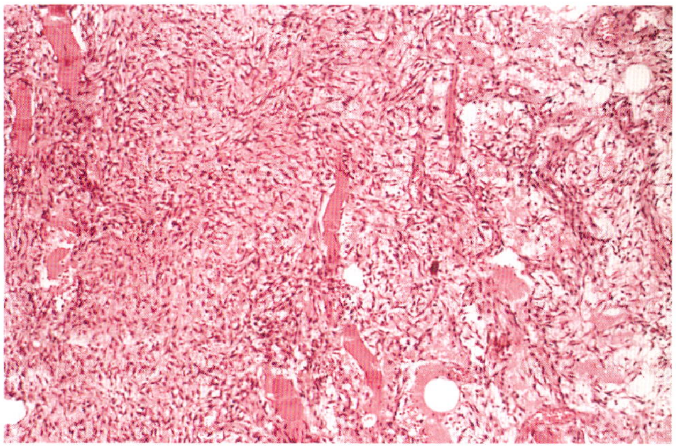

Figure 2-1. Early fracture callus with undifferentiated mesenchymal tissue. Note transition from striated muscle to undifferentiated mesenchymal tissue.

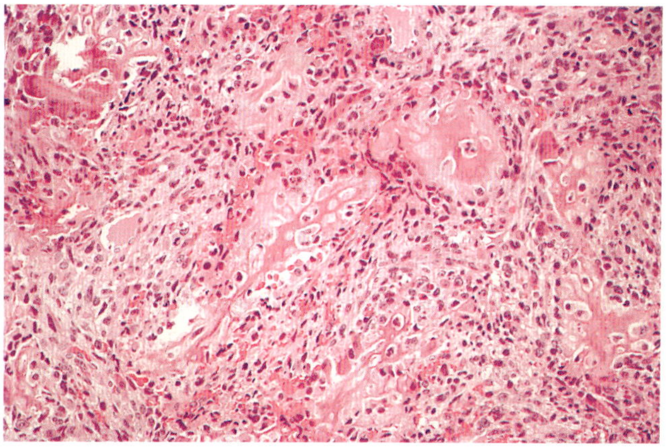

Figure 2-2. Osteosarcoma exhibiting numerous neoplastic mesenchymal cellular elements, fragments of primitive osteoid, and no apparent maturation process.

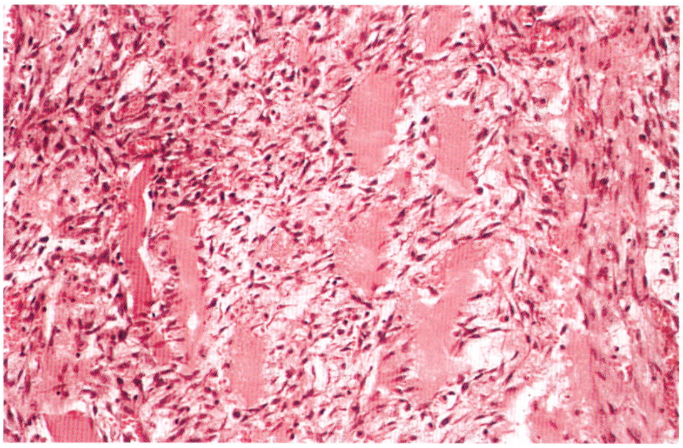

Figure 2-3. Early fracture callus. Striated muscle fibers undergoing degeneration and transition to undifferentiated mesenchymal tissue. Early fracture callus (Day 3).

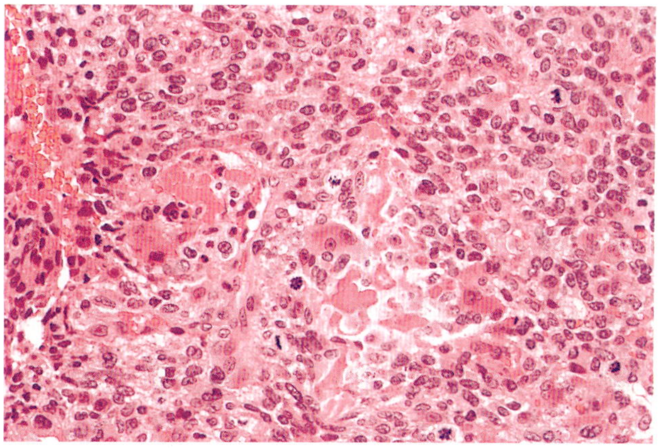

Figure 2-4. Osteosarcoma. Higher magnification exhibiting numerous neoplastic mesenchymal cellular elements. Fragments of primitive osteoid and no apparent maturation process.

Comment: It is often exceedingly difficult to differentiate early immature 3-day-old fracture callus from a neoplastic process. The pathologist must be aware of the possibility of a pathologic fracture in the midst of an otherwise benign lesion, and not confuse the early fracture callus with osteosarcoma. In the 3-day-old fracture callus this task may well be impossible.

ture field contributes to the formation of cartilage. The ability to transform the matrix of a cartilage cell into osteoid, retaining the nuclear structure of the cell, is a unique feature of fracture callus and has recently been confirmed experimentally.[1] This transformation can be easily demonstrated in all histologic sections of fracture, and identifiable ghost outlines of cartilaginous matrix usually persist in the maturing osteoid. The presence of this chondro-osseous transformation indicates the presence of fracture callus, regardless of the cellularity of the cartilage component (see Figures 3-2, 3-4, p. 43). One must remember that pathologic fracture, with chondro-osseous bone, can be present in the midst of a neoplastic process.

This maturation pattern is present in all reactive bone structures, be it fracture callus, periosteal reaction, or heterotopic ossification. In addition to cytologic analysis, to a large extent the differential diagnosis between a reactive process and a neoplasm is based on the presence or absence of this maturation process.

HETEROTOPIC OSSIFICATION

Heterotopic ossification differs from fracture callus throughout the absence of chondro-osseous bone. As a rule heterotopic ossification is composed of bone exclusively.

A characteristic typical pattern of maturation is noted. The peripheral portion of the heterotopic ossification is most mature, and sharply delineated from the surrounding tissue. As one approaches the center, the lesion becomes less mature, and can actually be confused with sarcoma. Characteristic zoning of the myositis ossificans is typical and serves to identify the lesion as a benign reactive entity.

Myositis ossificans is a soft tissue lesion, and may affect any mesenchymal component, not necessarily muscle. It may also secondarily attach to bone, and then offer difficulties in differentiating myositis ossificans from parosteal osteosarcoma or soft tissue osteosarcoma.[2,3] The most reliable radiographic feature is the presence of the most mature and heavily calcified tissue at the periphery, as opposed to the tumors, including surface sarcomas, which exhibit their least differentiated portion at the periphery of the calcified matrix.

REFERENCES

1. Hughes SS, Hicks DG, O'Keefe RJ, et al. Shared phenotypic expression of osteoblasts and chondrocytes in fracture callus. *J Bone Mineral Res* (accepted for publication) 1994.
2. Nuovo MA, Norman A, Chumas H, et al: Myositis ossificans with atypical clinical, radiographic, or pathologic findings: a review of 23 cases. *Skeletal Radiol* 21(2):88–101, 1992.
3. Schutte HE, van der Heul RO: Reactive mesenchymal proliferation. *J Belge Radiol* 75(4):297–302, 1992.

3

Osteoid Lesions

CENTRAL MEDULLARY OSTEOSARCOMA

Osteosarcoma is the most common primary malignant tumor of bone. It characteristically involves the metaphyseal portion of long bone, but may involve any bone of the body. There is rapid extension into diaphysis and epiphysis. Involvement of the growth plate is common. Although the tumor is most commonly seen in the second decade, osteosarcoma may occur at any age, any sex, and is frequently secondary to Paget's disease of bone in the older age population.

The radiographic appearance of the lesion usually presents as a poorly defined metaphyseal defect in long bone, either with moth-eaten or permeative destruction of the underlying bone. Extensive periosteal reaction, including streamer or onion-peel formation is often associated with the tumor. A Codman triangle indicates the rapid progression of the tumor. Matrix calcification of the tumor is not always present; some lesions are purely lytic. When matrix calcification is identifiable, it usually mimics trabeculae of bone, with a fine linear pattern rather than the flocculent calcification associated with cartilage.

In most instances, the histologic appearance does not present difficulty: one requires malignant neoplastic cells producing clearly identifiable osteoid. Numerous histologic patterns may exhibit variations of the theme. It is almost a matter of philosophy whether a given lesion which exhibits a predominant fibrous pattern and only minimal osteoid production should be called osteosarcoma or fibrosarcoma. Under current criteria, osteosarcoma is defined as a malignant neoplasm in which there is direct production of neoplastic osteoid by the tumor cell. Transition from cartilage or fibrous connective tissue to osteoid is not sufficient. It must be osteoid production by the malignant tumor cell. This is the current gold standard.

We have chosen to adopt the classification of osteosarcomas identified in the text by Mirra[1] with slight modification (Table 3-1). Since the advent of preoperative and postoperative chemotherapy, the histologic subtypes have assumed greater importance. Cartilage responds poorly or not at all to pre- or postoperative chemotherapy. An osteosarcoma with a large cartilaginous component will therefore not respond to adjuvant therapy as readily as the other subtypes, and some of the dense collagen-containing tumors also respond poorly. The histologic identification of the various subtypes therefore become a matter of some importance to the oncologist and surgeon. With more advanced techniques, one can look forward to prospective or interim evaluation of response to chemo- or radiation therapy, and correlate the response with the histologic subtype.[2,3]

Mixed Cell Pattern
Differential Diagnosis: Fracture Callus, Reactive Bone Formation

The histology exhibits a neoplasm with varying components of cartilaginous, fibrous, and osseous proliferation. The different patterns may be localized in different portions of the tumor. Adequate sampling assures the proper diagnosis. In many areas the type of osteoid produced by the tumor can vary from the large geographic

TABLE 3-1. Major Histologic Varieties of Primary Intramedullary and Juxtacortical Osteosarcoma

Dominant Histologic Patterns
I. Primary, solitary, high grade intramedullary osteosarcoma (predominant pattern approximately 80% of entire set of osteosarcomas)
A. Mixed patterns
B. Bone-rich or "sclerosing"
C. Cartilage-rich (chondrosarcoma-like)
D. Spindle cell–rich (fibrosarcoma-like)
E. Malignant histiocyte–rich (MFH-like)
F. Large vascular spaces or telangiectatic (ABC-like)
G. Small cell–rich (Ewing's sarcoma–like)
H. Benign giant cell–rich (giant cell tumor–like)
I. Epithelioid cell–rich (metastatic carcinoma–like)
II. Low grade intramedullary osteosarcoma (4–5% of entire set of osteosarcomas)
A. Intraosseous well-differentiated fibrous pattern
B. Osteoblastoma-like pattern
C. Chondromyxoid fibroma–like pattern
III. Juxtacortical tumors (7–10% of entire set of osteosarcomas)
A. Well-differentiated fibrous and osteoid pattern
B. Predominant cartilaginous pattern
C. Predominant fibrous pattern without osteoid formation
D. High grade surface osteosarcoma
IV. Osteocarcoma secondary to Paget's disease

MFH = malignant fibrous histiocytoma; ABC = aneurysmal bone cyst.
From Mirra JM, Picci P, Gold RH: *Bone Tumors. Clinical, Radiologic, and Pathologic Correlations.* Philadelphia, Lea and Febiger, 1989, p 254.

areas to small lacy deposits between the neoplastic cells. Large areas of malignant cells producing a fibrous pattern may accompany the production of the osteoid, neoplastic cartilage may be formed, and giant cells may be present in large numbers. The diagnosis must be based on neoplastic osteoid production by the tumor cell (Figures 3-1 to 3-6).

Sclerosing Pattern
Differential Diagnosis: Osteomyelitis, Paget's Disease

Osteosarcoma with a sclerosing pattern is readily evident on radiographic analysis, with almost complete "white-out" of the affected bone. The histologic section does not look particularly different from any other mixed pattern of osteosarcoma, but because of its extensive calcification, sections may require extensive additional decalcification. Neoplastic cells producing the osteoid are usually found thoughout the lesion, but can be easily identified at the advancing margin of such a tumor.

The differential diagnosis includes any sclerosing process within bone. Osteoma consists of masses of bone with little of any cellular component. Frequently, osteomyelitis will heal with the formation of large areas of reactive and sclerotic bone, exhibiting numerous reversal lines. Normal osteoblasts are present.

Paget's disease may form large areas of sclerosing bone, and replacement of the marrow by fibrous connective tissue is a uniform feature of active Paget's disease. Atypical osteoclasts are present. Usually the radiographic analysis is fairly straightforward, but occasionally small foci of asymptomatic Paget's disease may be confused with a neoplastic process. One must not forget that Paget's disease itself may lead to malignant transformation (see differential diagnosis of sarcoma in Paget's disease (Figures 3-9, 3-10, 3-26, 3-27).

The mere presence of large amounts of sclerosing heavily calcified bone, without the cellular pleomorphism or neoplastic cells producing osteoid, *is not a feature* of osteosarcoma (Figures 3-7 to 3-11).

Cartilage Predominant
Differential Diagnosis: Chondroma, Chondrosarcoma, Fracture Callus with Extensive Cartilage

There are many osteosarcomas in which 70–90% of the tumor consists of neoplastic cartilage. These in turn may produce bone. A cartilage tumor producing osteoid via cartilage precursor is not considered an osteosarcoma. The definition of osteosarcoma depends upon a focus of neoplastic cells directly producing identifiable osteoid. The remainder of the tumor may have large quantities of cartilage, but the identification of the small focus of osteoid production by the tumor cell is essential to identify cartilage-predominant osteosarcoma.

At times the presence of immature fracture callus with extensive cartilage is a challenge. One must be careful not to confuse the cartilage of fracture callus with any neoplastic process, either chondrosarcoma or cartilage-predominant osteosarcoma. The maturation process is usually a reliable feature. While fracture callus can exhibit areas with extensive hypercellularity of the cartilaginous component, there usually is no hyperchromatism, the cells are confined to the lacunar space, and there is no mitotic activity. The presence of chondro-osseous bone is the diagnostic hallmark of fracture (Figure 3-12 to 3-15).

MATURING FRACTURE CALLUS VERSUS OSTEOSARCOMA, MIXED PATTERN

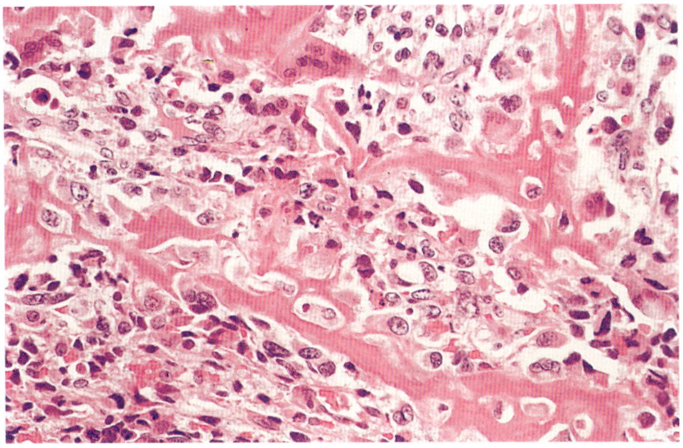

Figure 3-1. Osteosarcoma. Higher magnification of osteoid formation by a neoplasm. In the differential diagnosis of osteoid versus fibrous connective tissue, one must look for the lacunar space with the entrapped osteocyte as opposed to the spindled fibroblast seen in a fibrous lesion. In addition, osteoblasts line up along the edge of a fragment of osteoid rather than forming a spindled nucleus in the center of the fiber. Note the presence of osteoclasts, indicating the presence of calcified material capable of being resorbed.

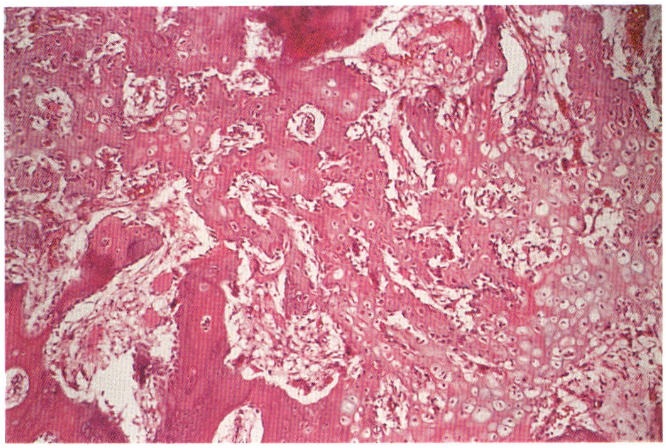

Figure 3-2. Maturing fracture callus. Note chondro-osseous bone, i.e., transformation of cartilage to osteoid matrix without change of nuclei. Notice maturation of connective tissue adjacent to the bone fragments.

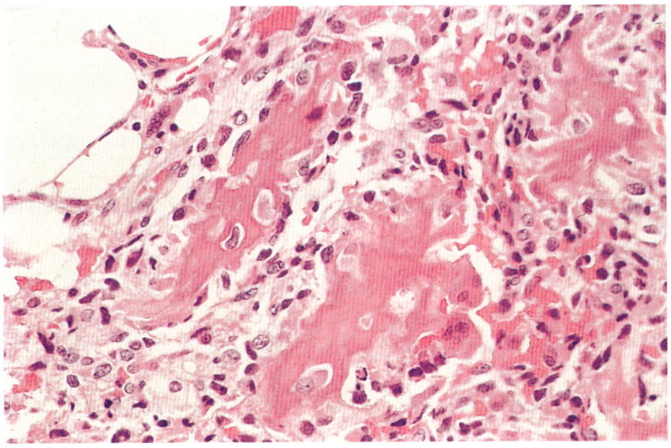

Figure 3-3. Osteosarcoma. Primitive osteoid and a highly cellular matrix exhibiting variation in size, shape, and staining of the osteoblastic nuclei.

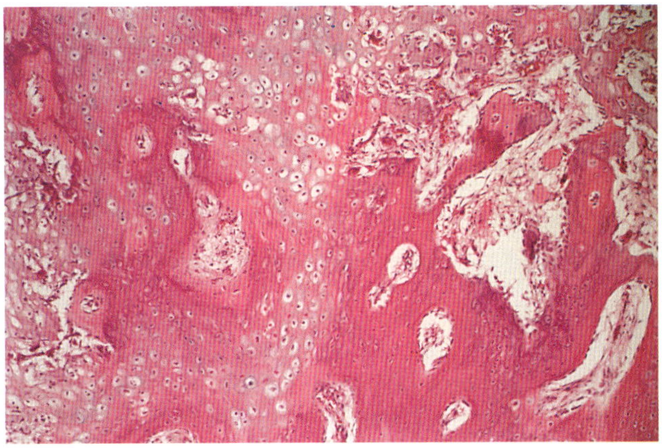

Figure 3-4. Fracture callus. Note the highly cellular cartilage undergoing transition to osteoid without abutment. Note maturation of connective tissue adjacent to the osteoblastic rim of the more mature bone fragments. Also note the residual chondroid structure in the more mature bone on the lower right-hand side of the picture.

Comment: The presence of chondro-osseous bone is a reliable indicator that the lesion contains components of a fracture. In this particular group of illustrations, there is evidence of a maturation pattern which again attests to the reactive nature of that field. The absence of both chondro-osseous bone and maturation process indicates a neoplastic process.

OSTEOSARCOMA

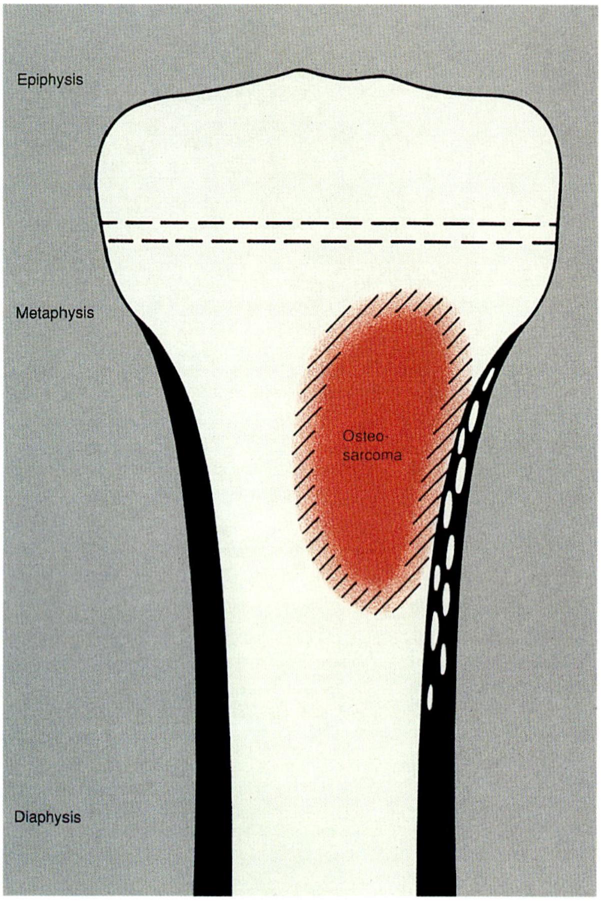

Figure 3-5. Radiographic demonstration of osteosarcoma. The lesion is usually metaphyseal, with poorly defined margins. It may have a moth-eaten, but more frequently, a permeative pattern through the adjacent trabecular and cortical bone. There may be a periosteal reaction, and if it is present, it is the rapidly destructive pattern, such as a Codman triangle, hair-on-end or lamellated proliferation.

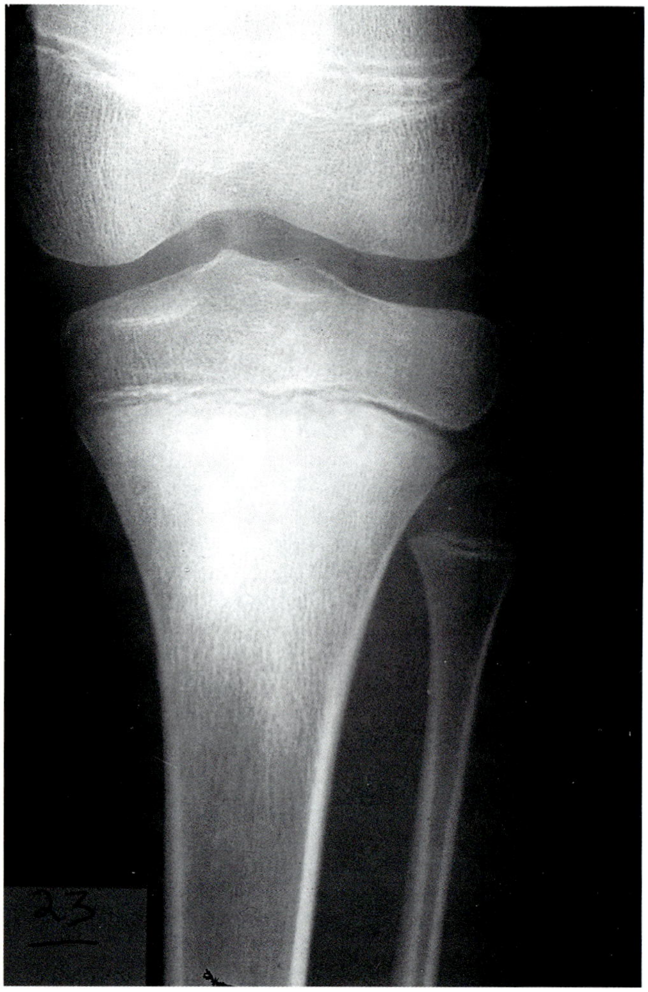

Figure 3-6. X-ray of patient with osteosarcoma. Notice metaphyseal location, poorly defined permeative growth, matrix calcification with a linear spiculed pattern. In this particular example there is no periosteal reaction.

DIFFERENTIAL DIAGNOSIS OF LESIONS WITH SCLEROSIS

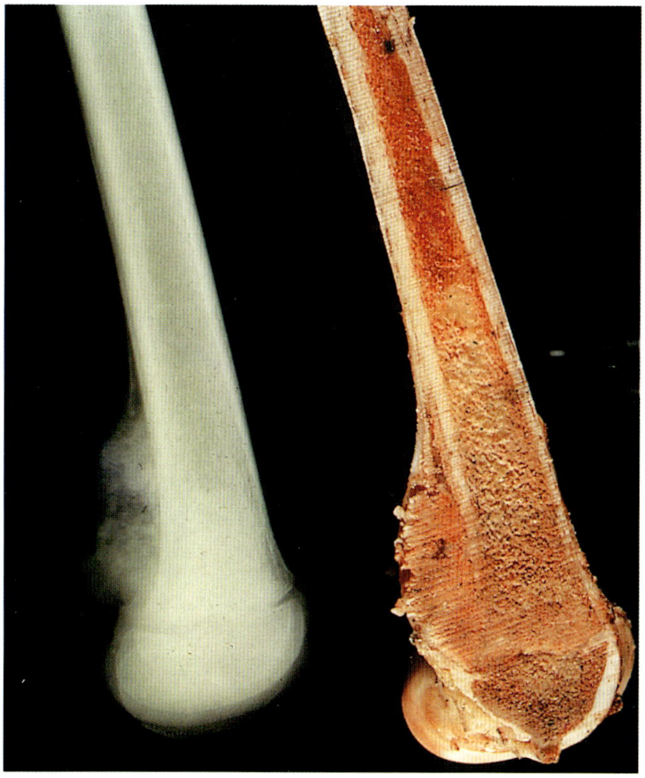

Figure 3-7. Specimen x-ray and corresponding specimen from a 14-year-old patient with osteosarcoma. Note the extension of the sarcoma across the growth plate into the epiphysis (not identified on plain film), extension into diaphysis, Codman triangle, and extension into soft tissue.

Spindle Cell–Rich Sarcoma
Differential Diagnosis: Fibrous Dysplasia, Nonossifying Fibroma with Bone Formation, Malignant Fibrous Histiocytoma, Osteomyelitis, Osteofibrous Dysplasia (ossifying fibroma)

The osteosarcoma which produces a spindled stroma may be confused with a malignant fibrous histiocytoma (MFH) or fibrosarcoma. While there is some controversy, it is our belief that a malignant fibrous histiocytoma does not produce any neoplastic osteoid. If a tumor produces even minute amounts of osteoid, it is classified as an osteosarcoma with a predominant spindle cell pattern. The usual rules of neoplasia apply: there must be pleomorphism, hyperchromatism, and significant mitotic activity. The tumor cell must produce neoplastic osteoid to be classified as osteosarcoma.

In the differential diagnosis one must consider fibrous dysplasia. Fibrous dysplasia is always characterized by proliferation of spindled collagen, producing cells with direct transition to immature bony trabeculae. As opposed to the MFH-like osteosarcoma, fibrous dysplasia produces uniform, evenly spaced bony trabeculae as the lesion matures. In the sarcoma there may be large areas where there is no bone production at all. Fibrous dysplasia is a slow growing process, expanding the bone, without extending into the adjacent soft tissue. On the other hand, a sarcoma with spindled components often breaks through the cortex into adjacent soft tissue.

The nonossifying fibroma normally heals with the production of bone, and indeed, that is the evolution of most nonossifying fibromas. The formation of bone is accompanied by benign xanthomatous elements, and undergoes an intermediate stage of calcification before there is actual bone formation. The bone that is formed may be immature, but does not exhibit any histologic features of malignancy.

Osteomyelitis in its healing stage may have a large fibrous component, and there may even be some mild variation in cell size and shape. However, the cellular features of malignancy are absent. In addition, the bone that is formed is appositional normal bone, adding to the thickness of preexisting trabeculae. Thus, numerous reversal lines are identified, and under polarized light the bony trabeculae exhibit a lamellar pattern.

Osteofibrous dysplasia is an intracortical lesion. It may exhibit fibrous proliferation, bone formation with plump osteoblasts lining the trabeculae of bone, but there should be no significant pleomorphism or mitotic activity. The intracortical osteofibrous dysplasia is precisely that: a lesion confined to the cortex. It may be difficult to demonstrate the intracortical location on the basis of isolated radiographs, and multiple views and additional studies may be required. Over 90% of the

DIFFERENTIAL DIAGNOSIS OF LESIONS WITH SCLEROSIS

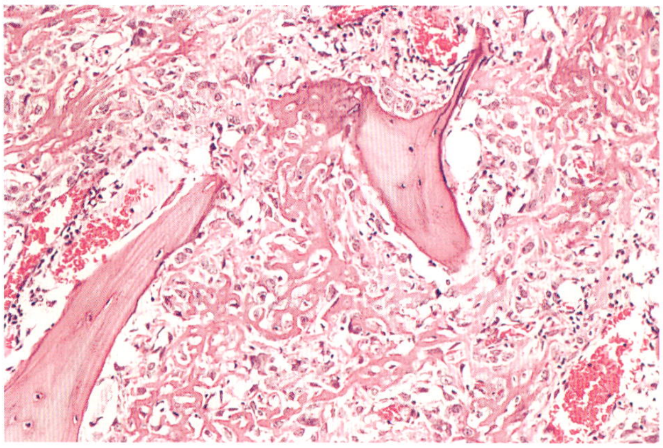

Figure 3-8. Sclerosing osteosarcoma. Extensive osteoid production filling the medullary space between trabeculae of mature bone. This pattern is diagnostic of osteosarcoma, and there really is no acceptable differential diagnosis.

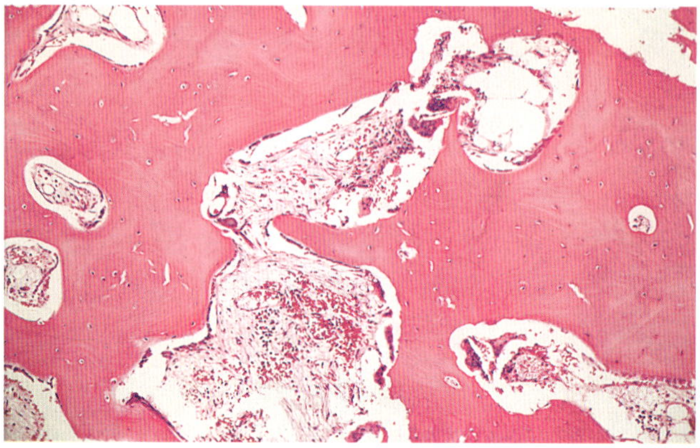

Figure 3-9. Paget's disease. Lamellar bone formation with extensive abnormal osteoclastic and osteoblastic activity. Note the "killer osteoclasts," i.e., numerous large osteoclasts with an abnormally large number of nuclei. In addition to the abnormal osteoclasts, there are numerous osteoblasts laying down pagetoid bone, and replacement of the normal fatty marrow by fibrous connective tissue. The mosaic of Paget's is not clearly visible on this section due to light staining with hematoxylin.

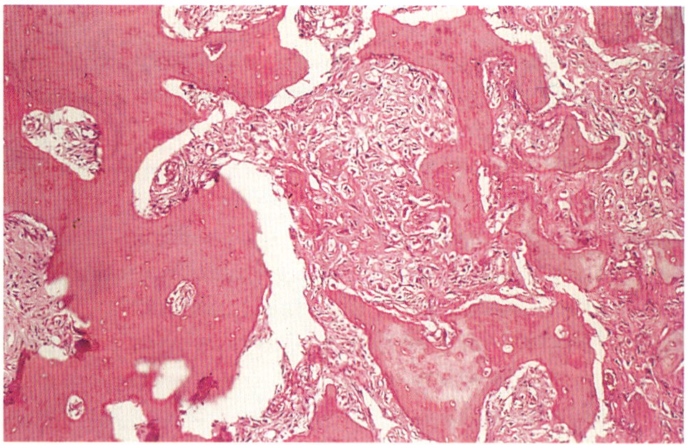

Figure 3-10. Sarcoma arising in Paget's disease. The patient had full-fledged Paget's disease. A cellular sarcomatous pattern is present between the residual pagetoid trabeculae.

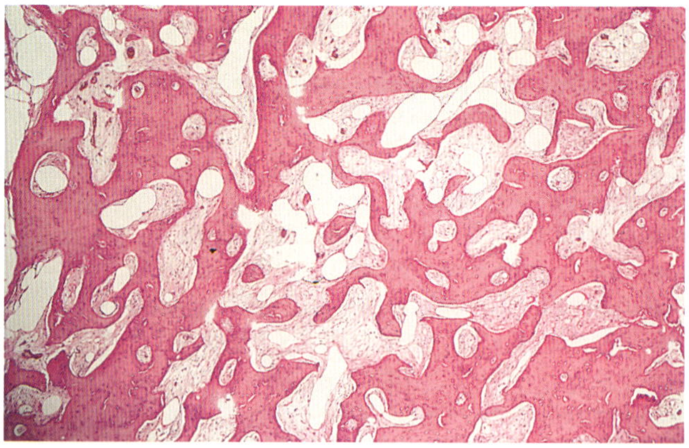

Figure 3-11. Reactive bone formation in chronic osteomyelitis. One should not forget that the scar tissue of bone is bone. When an osteomyelitis heals, there is a tendency for excessive bone formation, replacement of the marrow by fibrous connective tissue, and numerous sinusoidal vascular spaces, consistent with the new bone formation. No osteoclasts are visible, although there are some Howship lacunae indicating resorption and remodeling of the bone. The fibrous connective tissue is loose, edematous, and even at the low power magnification there does not appear to be any evidence of a neoplastic process.

DIFFERENTIAL DIAGNOSIS OF OSTEOID LESIONS WITH EXTENSIVE CARTILAGE

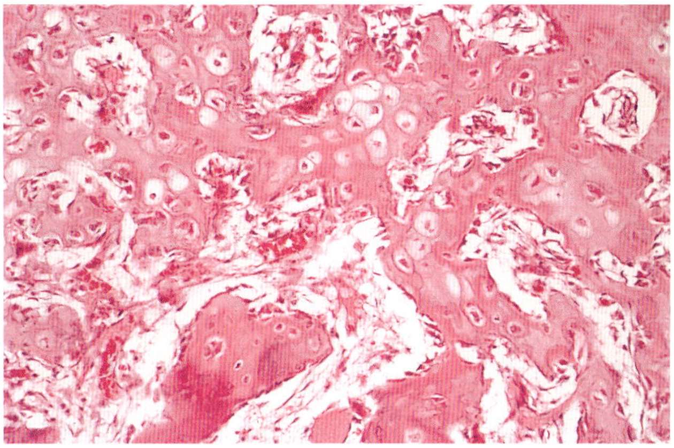

Figure 3-12. Maturing fracture callus demonstrating chondro-osseous bone, maturation of bony trabeculae and loss of cellular material in the spaces between the bony elements. Excessive vascularity (transition to sinusoidal phase) is evident.

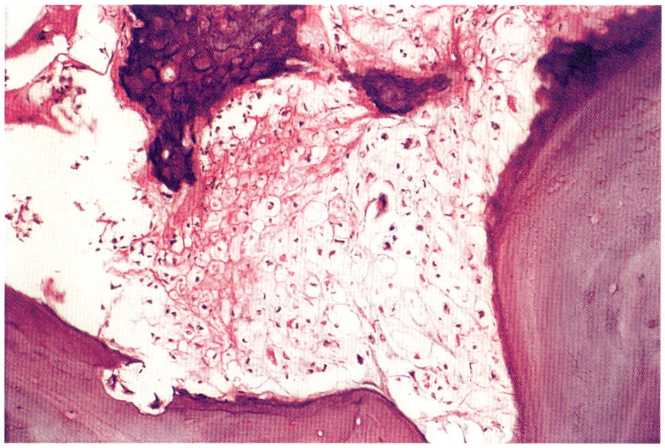

Figure 3-13. Clearly identifiable cartilage differentiation by an intraosseous neoplasm with secondary calcification.

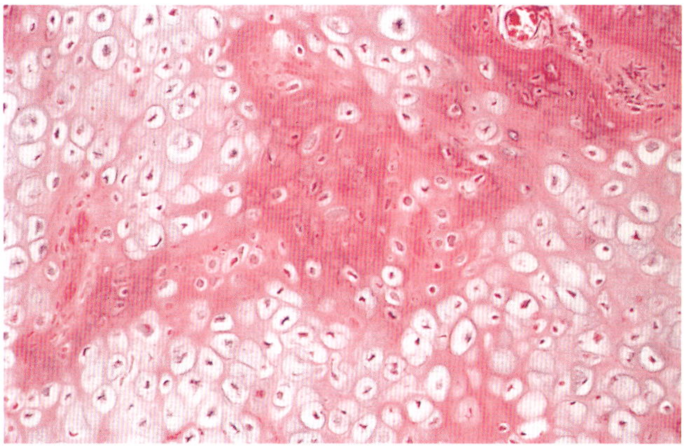

Figure 3-14. Fracture callus. Chondro-osseous bone exhibiting cellular cartilaginous component of the fracture undergoing transition to osteoid without loss of nuclear material. Chondro-osseous bone is always found in a fracture. It should not be confused with a chondroid neoplasm.

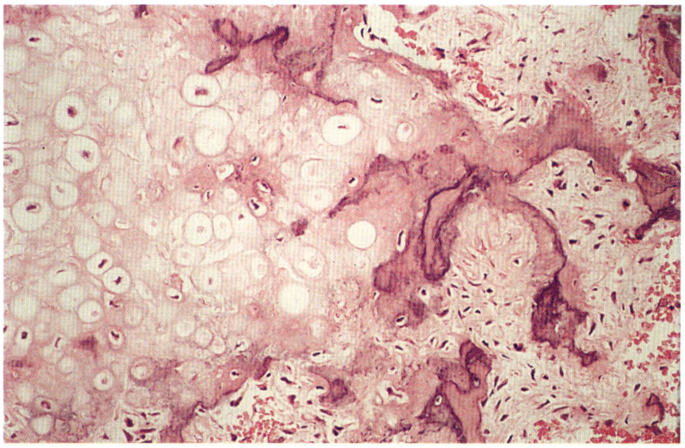

Figure 3-15. Osteosarcoma with prominent cartilage component. Note the neoplastic cartilage proliferation, similar to that found in fracture callus, but there is no evidence of chondro-osseous transformation and the lesion abuts against the adjacent, moderately pleomorphic stroma.

DIFFERENTIAL DIAGNOSIS OF OSTEOID LESIONS WITH EXTENSIVE FIBROUS COMPONENT

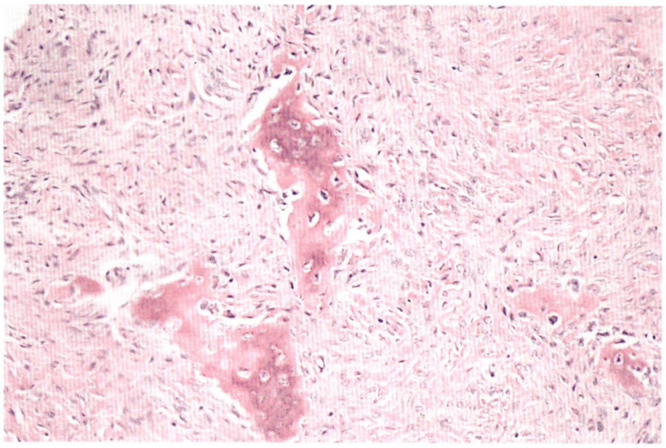

Figure 3-16. Well-differentiated osteosarcoma forming neoplastic bone in the midst of what appears to be benign fibrous proliferation. One must be careful not to confuse this type of proliferation with fibrous dysplasia. As opposed to fibrous dysplasia, bone formation is irregular, focal, with some variation in maturation.

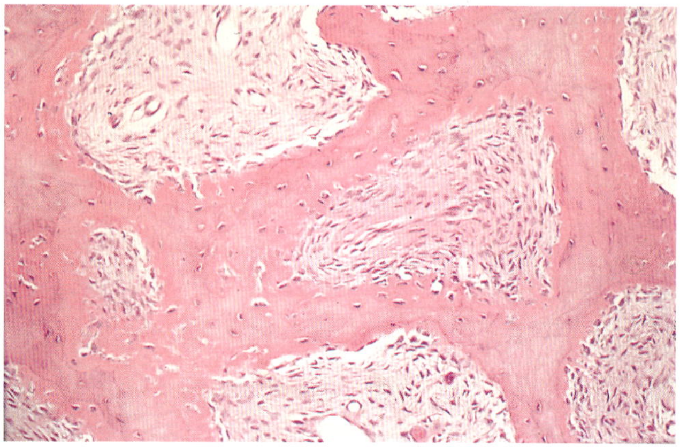

Figure 3-17. Fibrous dysplasia, immature bone, relatively mature and uniform fibrous elements. No rimming osteoblasts. The cells that line up along the osteoblastic seam are flattened, and similar to the fibrous elements within the lesion itself.

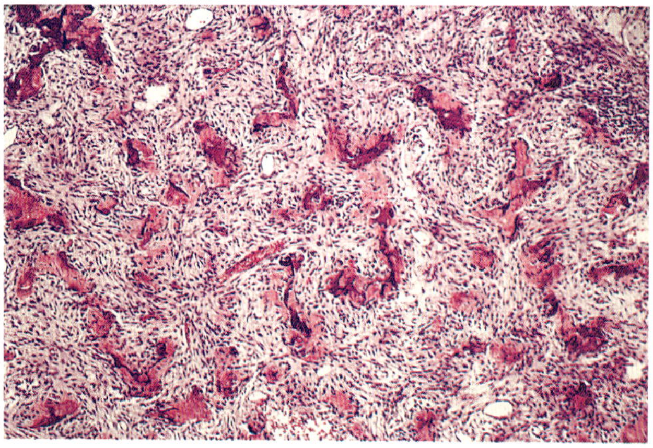

Figure 3-18. Nonossifying fibroma undergoing calcification and secondary ossification. Note the xanthomatous component, a spindled fibrous component, and ossification via calcification.

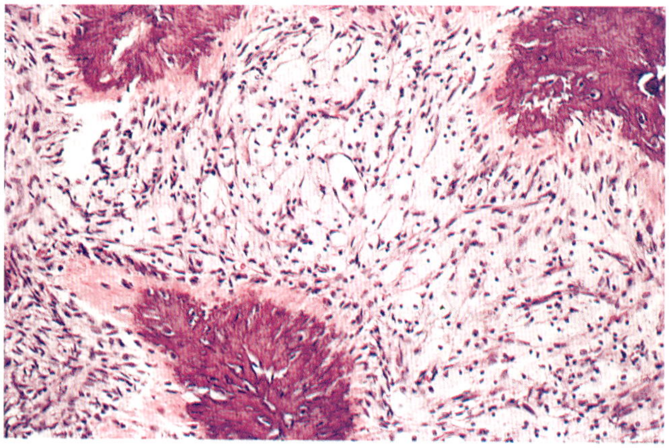

Figure 3-19. Nonossifying fibroma undergoing calcification and secondary ossification. The diagnostic features of a nonossifying fibroma are present, and include a fibrous proliferation with storiform pattern, and numerous xanthoma cells.

DIFFERENTIAL DIAGNOSIS OF OSTEOID LESIONS WITH EXTENSIVE FIBROUS COMPONENT

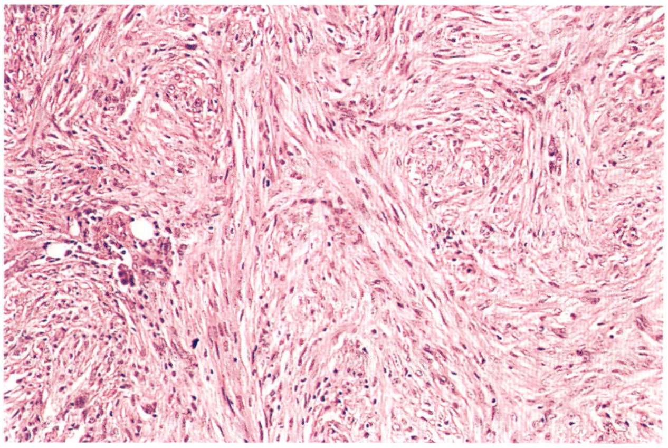

Figure 3-20. Osteosarcoma with predominant malignant fibrous histiocytoma pattern. In this illustration, by itself, one could not make a diagnosis of osteosarcoma as there is no neoplastic osteoid formation. The storiform pattern is characteristic of a malignant fibrous histiocytoma. Nuclear pleomorphism and mitotic activity are noted.

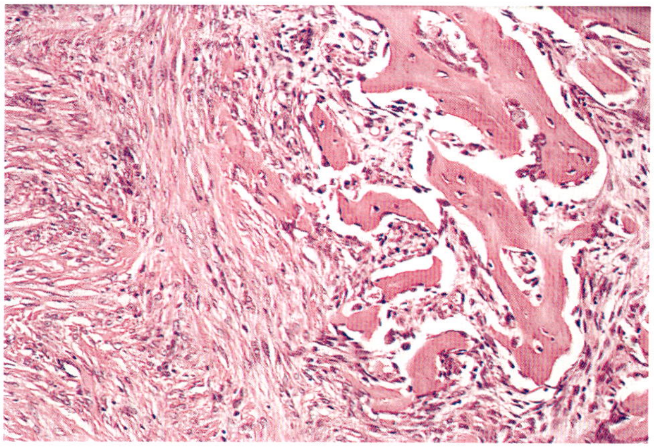

Figure 3-21. Osteosarcoma with predominant malignant fibrous histiocytoma pattern. In the midst of this MFH-like pattern there are focal areas of neoplastic osteoid formation. Even though these areas may be relatively minor, the formation of osteoid by the tumor cell establishes the diagnosis of osteosarcoma.

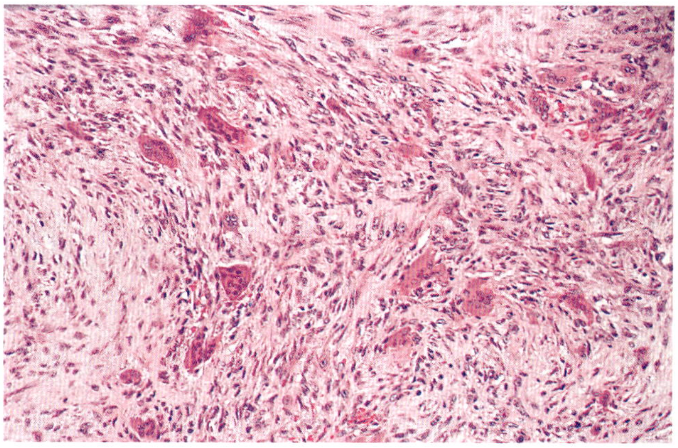

Figure 3-22. Malignant fibrous histiocytoma. A noncalcifying fibrous proliferation with characteristic storiform proliferation associated with numerous giant cells. In this illustration the pleomorphism of the cells is minimal, the storiform pattern is apparent, the lesion could easily be confused with a benign nonossifying fibroma.

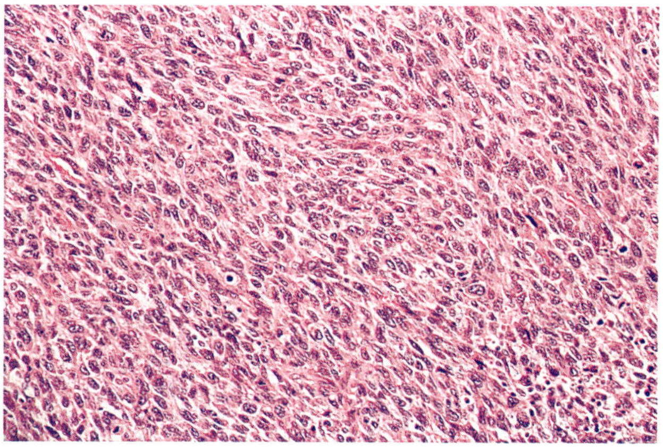

Figure 3-23. Other fields from the same tumor (*above*) exhibit this highly cellular tumor with plump epithelioid cells forming a collagen fiber pattern and numerous mitotic figures. Areas of malignant fibrous histiocytoma can vary, and one must be sure to examine the entire field establishing the diagnosis on the characteristic areas which are usually found in the advancing margin of the tumor. The malignant fibrous histiocytoma does not calcify, and does not form bone or cartilage.

DIFFERENTIAL DIAGNOSIS OF OSTEOID LESIONS WITH EXTENSIVE FIBROUS COMPONENT

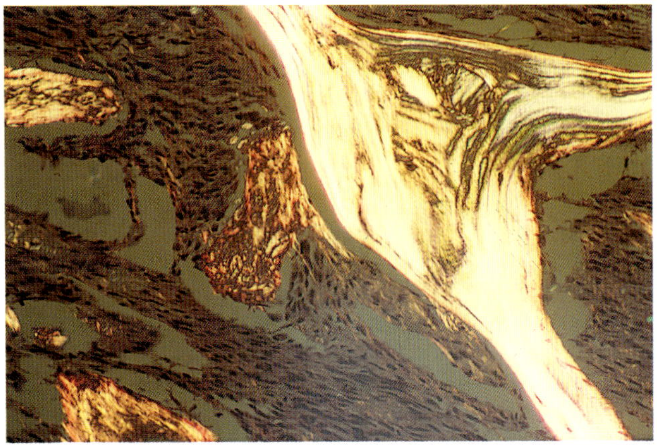

Figure 3-24. Osteosarcoma. Histologic examination of osteosarcoma infiltrating trabecular bone. The residual trabecular bone exhibits a well-differentiated lamellar pattern under polarized light, whereas the neoplastic bone exhibits a woven pattern.

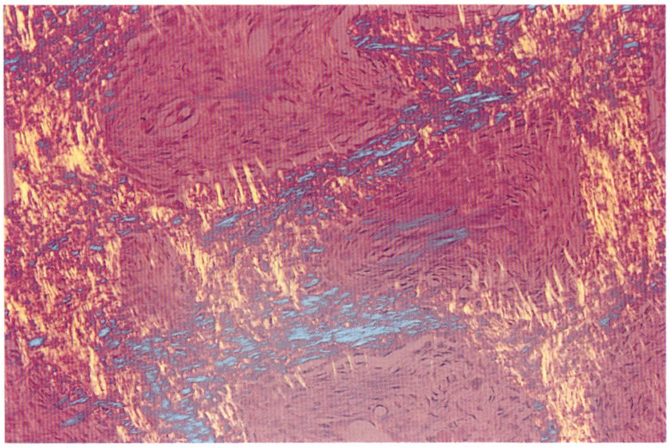

Figure 3-25. Fibrous dysplasia. Examination under polarized light exhibits a uniform woven pattern throughout all elements of fibrous dysplasia.

lesions are found in the tibia or fibula, although they may be multiple in those bones (Figures 3-16 to 3-28).

Telangiectatic Osteosarcoma
Differential Diagnosis: Aneurysmal Bone Cyst

The pattern is one of high grade intramedullary osteosarcoma with prominent vascular component and little bone formation. The vascular spaces are spread throughout the tumor, and there is no identifiable endothelial lining in the vascular structures, but rather lakes of blood with adjacent tumor cells. Radiographically these lesions are lytic. Histologic examination often requires extensive search for osteoid formation by the tumor. The stroma is characterized by numerous pleomorphic hyperchromatic cells.

The differential diagnosis includes the aneurysmal bone cyst. Unless it is secondary to a malignant process, the aneurysmal bone cyst is a benign lesion and will have a sharply circumscribed margin with expansion of the cortex. The vascular spaces are similar to the sarcoma, with stromal cells, no identifiable vessel lining, and numerous giant cells in the cellular tissue adjacent to the blood space, but the aneurysmal bone cyst does not contain pleomorphic or hyperchromatic cells; the histologic appearance of the tissue is always benign. There is usually a small, thin, bony rim at the edge of the aneurysmal cyst, composed of unremarkable reactive bone (Figures 3-29 to 3-32).

Small Cell Osteosarcoma
Differential Diagnosis: Ewing's Sarcoma, Lymphoma, Metastatic Neuroendocrine Tumor

Small cell, round cell (WHO) or mesenchymal osteosarcoma is a rare variant. All reported cases show some osteoid formation. The tumor can be confused with the round cell tumors or metastatic lesions (see Chapter 7, Round Cell Lesions); adequate sampling is required to identify the osteoid producing cells[4,5] (See Figures 7-1 to 7-4, differential diagnosis of round cell lesions, p. 104).

Giant Cell–Rich
Differential Diagnosis: giant cell tumor, osteoblastoma with numerous giant cells

All lesions of the skeleton exhibit varying components of osteoclastic derivatives, i.e., giant cells. In some instances the giant cells actually are either the neoplastic component itself (see Chapter 6, Giant Cell Tumor of Bone, p 97) or a predominant feature of the neoplasm (see Chondroblastoma, Chapter 4, p 75). If there is extensive osteoid formation one is not dealing with a giant cell tumor, but rather with an osteoblastoma or an osteosarcoma with a large giant cell component. The giant cells themselves may be benign or malignant; their presence does not establish a particular diagnosis, but rather one must look for osteoid formation by the tumor. Giant

DIFFERENTIAL DIAGNOSIS OF OSTEOID LESIONS WITH EXTENSIVE FIBROUS COMPONENT (PAGET'S DISEASE, WITH SARCOMA, AND OSTEOFIBROUS DYSPLASIA)

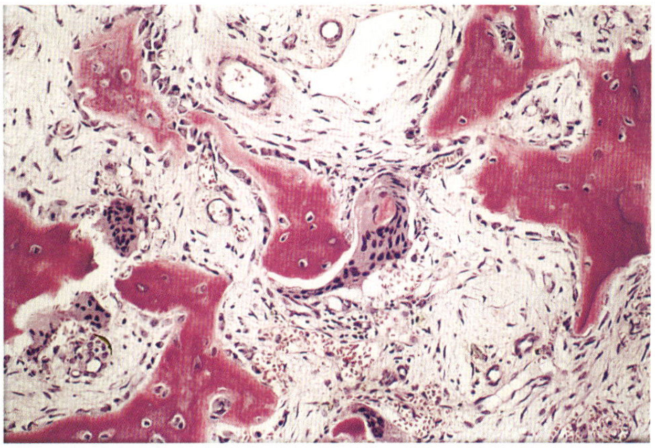

Figure 3-26. Paget's disease. Trabeculae of bone exhibiting both osteoclastic and osteoblastic activity on the same osteoblastic seam. Fibrous replacement of marrow. Clusters of inflammatory cells (chiefly lymphocytes), "killer osteoclasts": unusually large osteoclasts with numerous nuclei. This photograph illustrates the early lytic phase of Paget's disease.

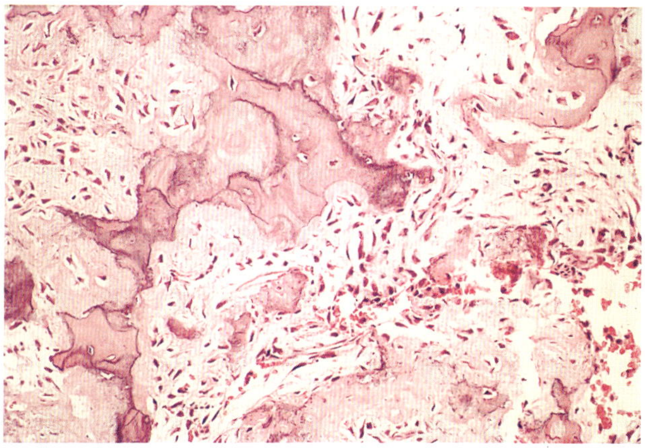

Figure 3-27. Paget's disease with sarcomatous transformation. Compare to Figure 3-26 and note the difference in the fibrous connective tissue stroma. In this particular illustration the fibrous connective tissue exhibits marked pleomorphism, a collagen spindled pattern, and mitotic activity as well as neoplastic osteoid formation.

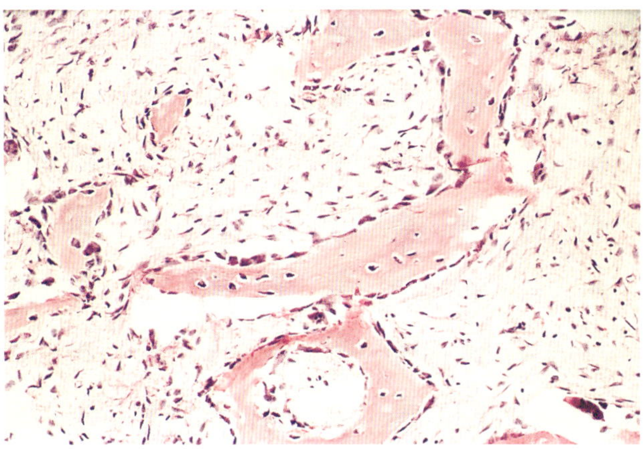

Figure 3-28. Osteofibrous dysplasia. Formation of osteoid with rimming osteoblasts. The remainder of the tissue is fibrous connective tissue with uniform fibroblasts. There is a superficial similarity to fibrous dysplasia, but the osteoblastic rimming is prominent.

cells may predominate in benign osteoblastoma as well as in osteosarcoma.

The true giant cell tumor of bone may produce minute quantities of osteoid. It should never produce identifiable cartilage. The essential diagnostic feature of a giant cell tumor is the interchangeability of the stromal cell nucleus with the nucleus of the giant cell. Radiographically the giant cell tumor of bone is always lytic, and located near a growth plate (Figures 3-33 to 3-36).

Intraosseous Well-differentiated Osteosarcoma Differential Diagnosis: Fibrous Dysplasia, Nonossifying Fibroma, Healing Osteomyelitis, Paget's Disease

The intraosseous well-differentiated sarcoma is a variant which may be confused either with fibrous dysplasia, a nonossifying fibroma undergoing calcification and ultimate ossification, or the rare intracortical osteofibrous dysplasia.[6–8] The lesion usually grows more slowly than the usual osteosarcoma, and a search must be made for the neoplastic cellular elements producing osteoid. As opposed to fibrous dysplasia, the well-differentiated osteosarcoma may have areas in which residual trabecular bone is present within the lesion, and these will exhibit

DIFFERENTIAL DIAGNOSIS OF OSTEOID LESIONS WITH EXTENSIVE HEMORRHAGIC COMPONENT

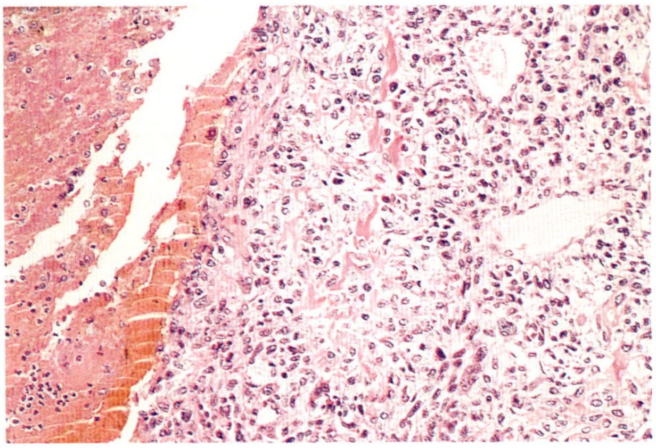

Figure 3-29. Telangiectatic pleomorphic osteolytic sarcoma. Higher magnification showing a moderately pleomorphic tumor producing neoplastic osteoid accompanied by large vascular spaces.

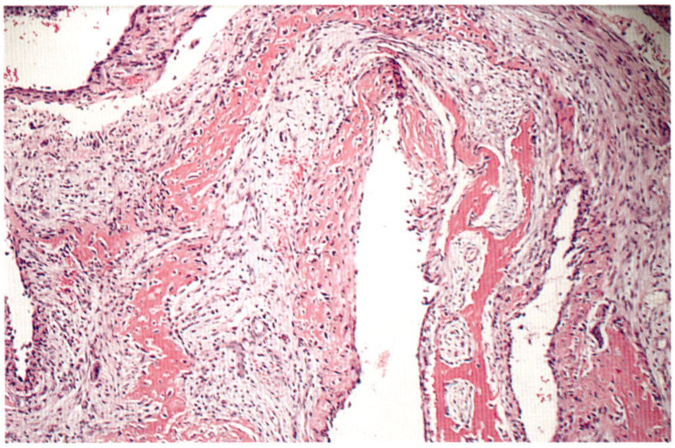

Figure 3-30. Aneurysmal bone cyst. The cavity does not contain a continuous endothelial lining surface. Scattered mesothelial cells are present at the surface. A bony rim is present beneath the cyst, composed of both primitive immature osteoid as well as more mature bone. The adjacent connective tissue is haphazard and contains scattered giant cells.

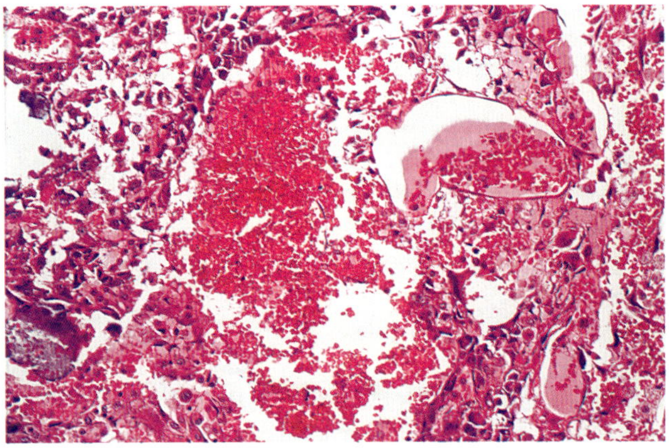

Figure 3-31. Telangiectatic pleomorphic osteolytic sarcoma, exhibiting markedly pleomorphic osteoblasts, with only isolated areas where osteoid is demonstrated. Numerous dilated vascular channels and hemorrhage within the tumor.

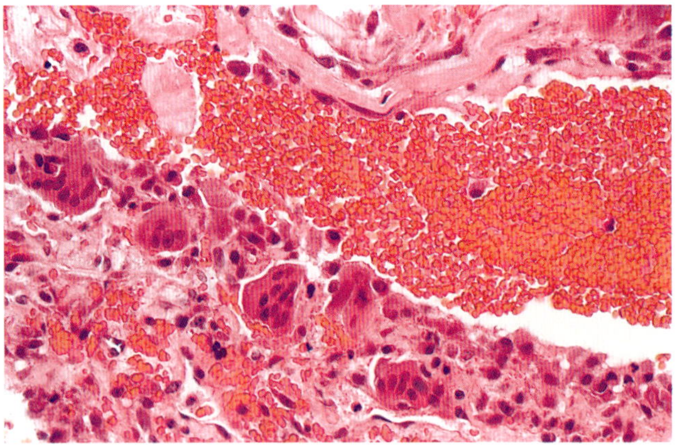

Figure 3-32. Aneurysmal bone cyst. The cavity is filled with red blood cells, there is no endothelial lining, numerous giant cells are present near the lumen of the cyst, some protruding into the lumen. The wall of the aneurysmal bone cyst contains unremarkable appearing connective tissue.

DIFFERENTIAL DIAGNOSIS OF OSTEOID LESIONS WITH NUMEROUS GIANT CELLS

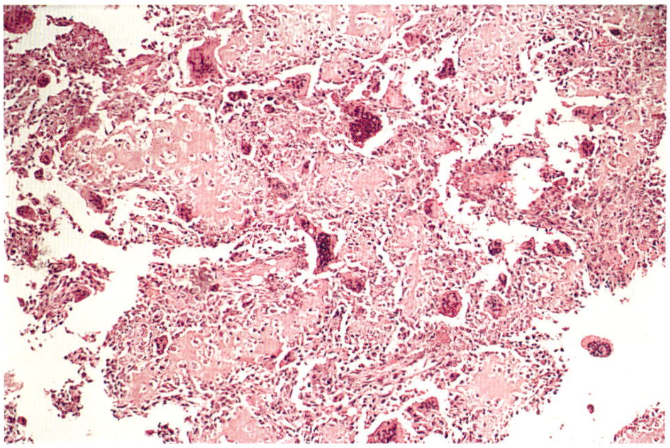

Figure 3-33. Giant cell–rich osteosarcoma. Note the production of neoplastic osteoid by the tumor. Despite the presence of numerous giant cells, this degree of osteoid production is not compatible with the diagnosis of giant cell tumor.

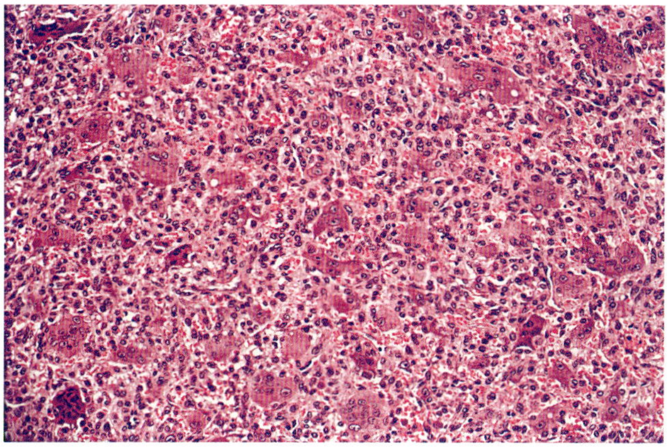

Figure 3-34. Giant cell tumor of bone. Numerous giant cells and stromal cells. The nuclei of the stromal cells can be placed within the giant cell and are interchangeable in size, configuration, and nuclear characteristics.

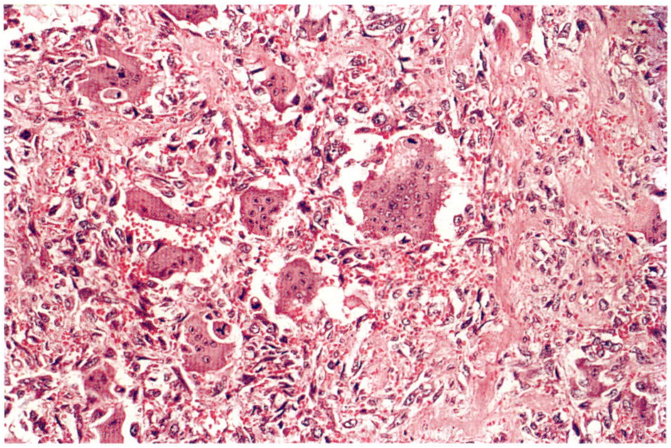

Figure 3-35. Osteosarcoma with numerous giant cells. The diagnosis of osteosarcoma must be based on the formation of neoplastic osteoid by the tumor cell. Numerous giant cells may accompany many lesions, including osteosarcoma.

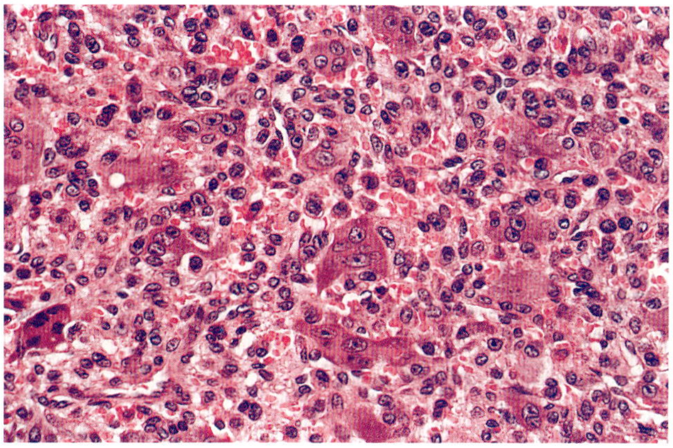

Figure 3-36. Higher magnification of Figure 3-34.

a lamellar pattern under polarized light (Figure 3-15). The newly formed neoplastic bone will show immature characteristics, i.e., woven bone.

In fibrous dysplasia the pattern of ossification is fairly uniform throughout the lesion, maturing at the same rate throughout. In an osteosarcoma there may be large areas where there is no osteoid production at all. Plump osteoblasts rimming bony trabeculae are never a feature of fibrous dysplasia, although occasional spindled cells mimicking osteoblasts and lining up adjacent to trabeculae may be identified (Figures 3-37 to 3-39).

Osteoblastoma-like Pattern Differential Diagnosis: Osteoblastoma, Osteoid Osteoma

Osteosarcomas forming clusters of well-differentiated osteoblasts with only minimal pleomorphism and mitotic activity are difficult to differentiate from the classical osteoblastoma.[9,10] The presence of fine linear calcification (the lacy osteoid pattern), coupled with the

DIFFERENTIAL DIAGNOSIS OF OSTEOID LESIONS WITH BENIGN-APPEARING FIBROUS COMPONENT

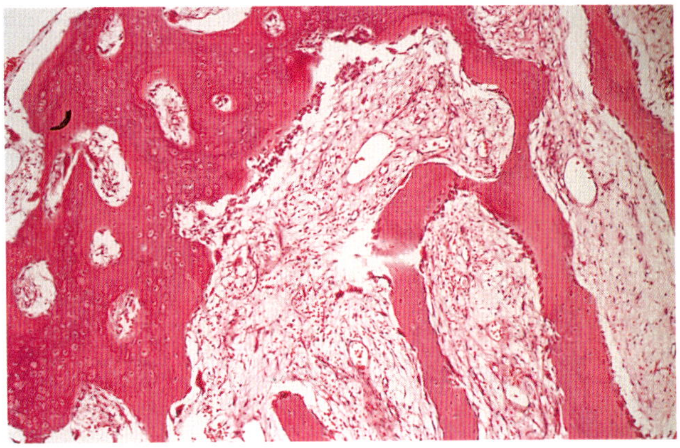

Figure 3-37. Healing fracture. Residual chondro-osseous bone and a maturation process in the connective tissue elements between the trabeculae. Prominent osteoblastic rimming of bone is noted. A number of sinusoidal channels are evident, and as the fracture matures further, numerous additional sinusoidal channels will be formed.

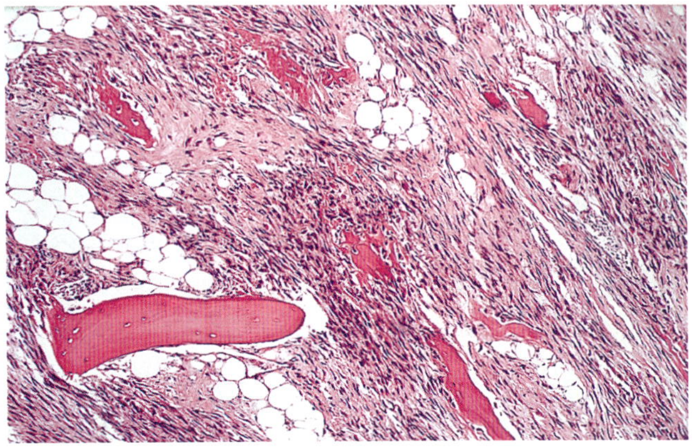

Figure 3-38. Osteosarcoma, spindled pattern. Note neoplastic formation of osteoid adjacent to residual trabecular bone. The invasion of the marrow cavity by this predominantly spindled neoplastic process is haphazard, and indicates a permeative destructive pattern.

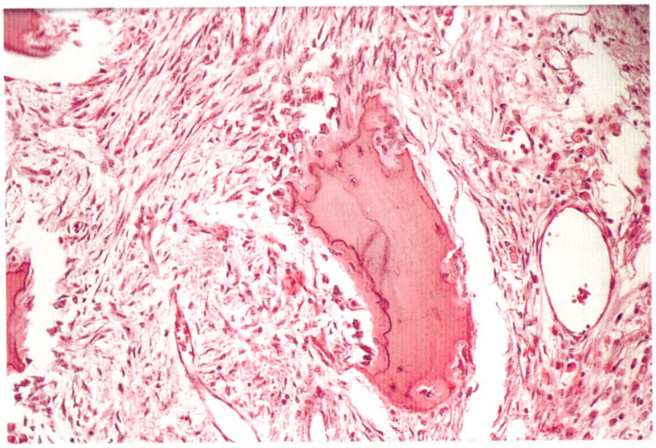

Figure 3-39. Osteomyelitis. Normal marrow has been replaced by fibrous connective tissue. Numerous Howship lacunae and reversal lines indicate active remodeling. An inflammatory infiltrate is identifiable within the connective tissue.

more aggressive radiographic appearance of these lesions leads to the diagnosis of osteosarcoma rather than osteoblastoma. In addition to the lacy osteoid, the tumor must present with a moderate degree of pleomorphism and abnormal mitotic figures. On permanent sections the differential diagnosis between the two entities is usually not difficult; difficulties may arise on frozen section, when the pathologist is tempted to make a diagnosis of osteoblastoma. One should not forget that an osteoblastoma is a benign lesion, and must have benign radiographic features, especially at the margin. Despite its lower biologic potential, the osteoblastoma-like osteosarcoma is not a benign lesion, will usually express itself by an infiltrative moth-eaten or permeative pattern, and will produce a periosteal reaction (Figures 3-40 to 3-49).

Chrondromyxoid Fibroma-like Pattern
Differential Diagnosis: Chondromyxoid Fibroma

The chondromyxoid fibroma-like pattern is similar to the osteoblastoma-like pattern: there is a superficial resemblance to a benign lesion, in this case, the chondromyxoid fibroma (CMF). However, the chondromyxoid fibroma does not produce neoplastic osteoid, and this variant of osteosarcoma does. In addition to discernible osteoid production by the tumor cell, the CMF-like osteosarcoma produces areas of myxoid matrix coupled with spindled tumor cells, areas of hypercellularity, and areas with giant cells, all of these features similar to the benign chondromyxoid fibroma. The differential diagnosis again depends upon the aggressive radiographic appearance, and the presence of clearly definable neoplastic osteoid production by the tumor cell, coupled with a moderate degree of pleomorphism and abnormal mitotic activity (see Figures 4-32, 4-33, p 76).

DIFFERENTIAL DIAGNOSIS, OSTEOID OSTEOMA, OSTEOBLASTOMA AND OSTEOSARCOMA

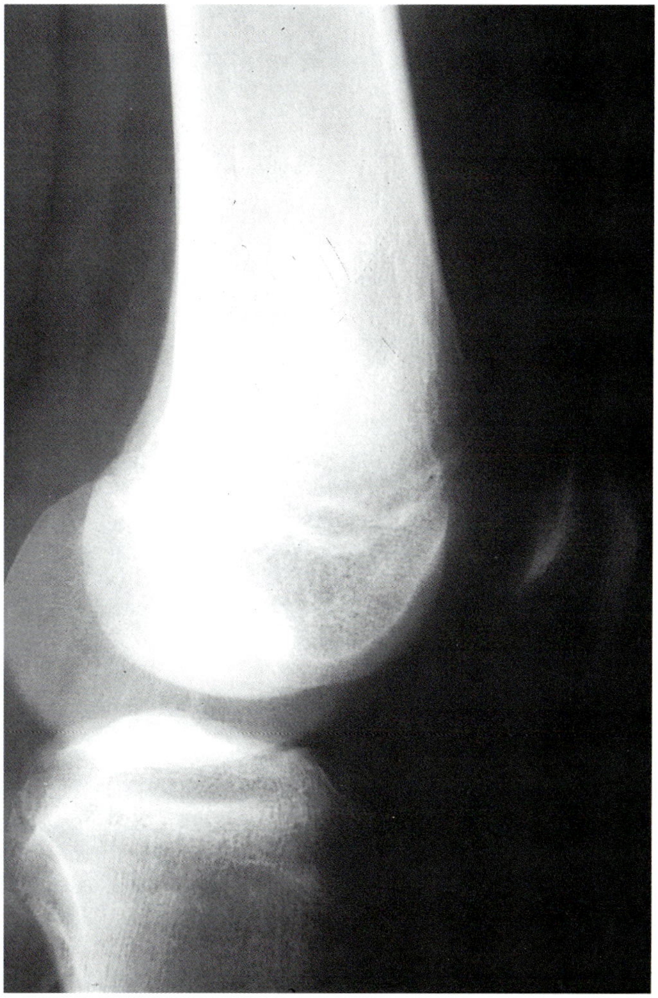

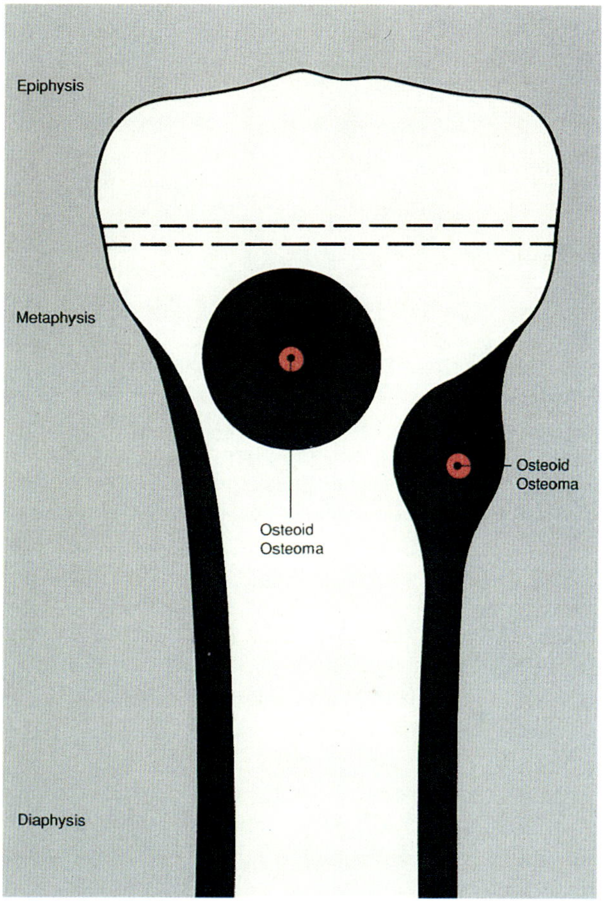

Figures 3-40, 3-41. The osteoid osteoma is a lytic process which evokes an unusual and excessive response on the part of the host bone. It may be found anywhere within the medullary cavity, intracortical or even intraperiosteal, and may involve any bone of the body. The nidus should not be more than 0.5 cm in diameter, although the reactive rim of bone around the nidus may be quite excessive.

DIFFERENTIAL DIAGNOSIS, OSTEOID OSTEOMA, OSTEOBLASTOMA AND OSTEOSARCOMA

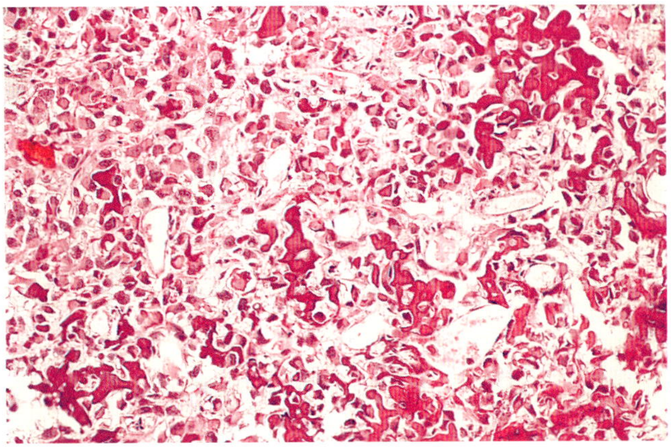

Figure 3-42. Osteoblastoma-like osteosarcoma. The lesion consists of numerous plump osteoblasts with the formation of prominent geographic osteoid. There is moderate pleomorphism of the osteoblast, but no abnormal mitotic figures are identified. The differential diagnosis includes osteoblastoma, and probably cannot be made on this particular illustration.

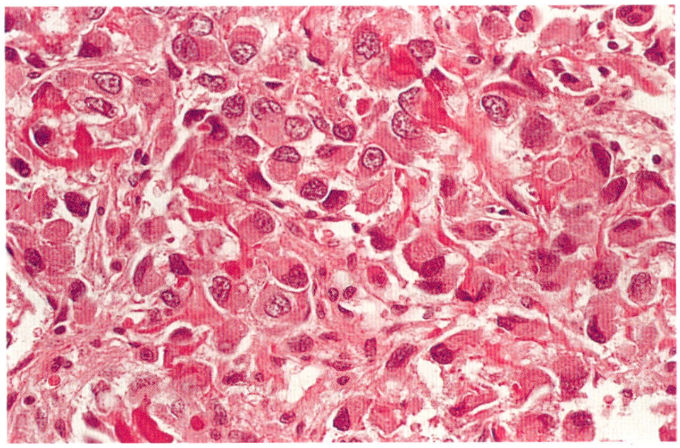

Figure 3-43. Higher magnification of Figure 3-48. Numerous osteoblasts, very prominent clear zones, but note the very thin lacy osteoid that is being produced by the tumor cell. An osteoblastoma should always produce large geographic areas of osteoid. When lacy osteoid of this nature is being produced by the tumor cell one should think of the osteoblastoma-like osteosarcoma, as in this particular patient.

Surface Osteosarcoma
Differential Diagnosis: Subungual Exostosis, Fibrous Dysplasia, Osteochondroma, Myositis Ossificans, Soft Tissue Sarcoma

Parosteal Juxtacortical Osteosarcoma. These tumors usually involve the tubular bones, most commonly the femur and tibia. The tumors originate on the periosteal surface and grow outward as well as indenting the underlying cortical surface. The lesion is characterized by slow growth, often many years.[11]

The radiographic features include a dense sclerotic mass attached to the outer surface of tubular bone, usually metaphyseal. There may be a thin zone of connective tissue separating portions of the tumor from the cortex. Periosteal new bone formation or a Codman triangle should not be a feature.

The histology of the lesion is often characterized by bland fibrous connective tissue. Foci of neoplastic osteoid formation are few and difficult to identify. The lesion is often confused with a benign entity (osteochondroma, fibrous dysplasia) but the exophytic growth pattern should exclude fibrous dysplasia, and the lack of marrow within the bony component should exclude osteochondroma. Careful search will find focal areas of increased cellularity, mitotic activity and pleomorphism, sufficient to justify the diagnosis of osteosarcoma. Occasional tumors exhibit high grade poorly differentiated neoplastic features.

The differential diagnosis includes myositis ossificans. Myositis ossificans occasionally becomes adherent to the cortical bone and exhibits histologic similarities to parosteal osteosarcoma. It should be remembered that the peripheral margin of a parosteal osteosarcoma is the least differentiated portion of the tumor, whereas myositis ossificans exhibits its most differentiated portion at the periphery with zones of more undifferentiated tissue closer to the center of the lesion. Ultimately a myositis ossificans will mature into normal bone and marrow (Figures 3-50 to 3-56).

Periosteal Osteosarcoma. The periosteal osteosarcoma is an entity described by Unni in 1976 to differentiate it from the conventional parosteal osteosarcoma.[12] It is usually a lytic scalloped lesion on the periosteal surface with a generous component of cartilaginous tissue. Neoplastic osteoid formation must be present[13] (Figure 3-57).

Juxtacortical (Periosteal) Chondroma and Chondrosarcoma. The juxtacortical (periosteal) chondromas and sarcomas are similar to the periosteal osteosarcoma in location and radiographic appearance. The essential difference is the absence of neoplastic osteoid formation by the juxtacortical chondroid tumors, whereas the periosteal osteosarcoma, while it may have extensive neo-

DIFFERENTIAL DIAGNOSIS, OSTEOID OSTEOMA, OSTEOBLASTOMA AND OSTEOSARCOMA

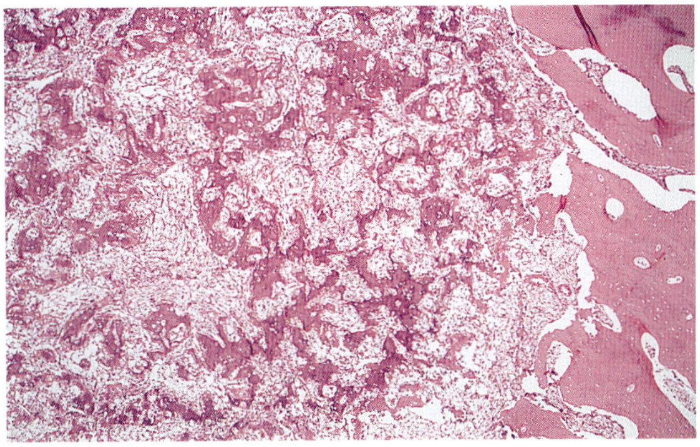

Figure 3-44. Osteoid osteoma. The nidus of an osteoid osteoma consists of tissue similar to osteoblastoma, but self-limiting, and characterized by an extensive rim of dense reactive bone at the edge rather than the thin shell as is present in the osteoblastoma.

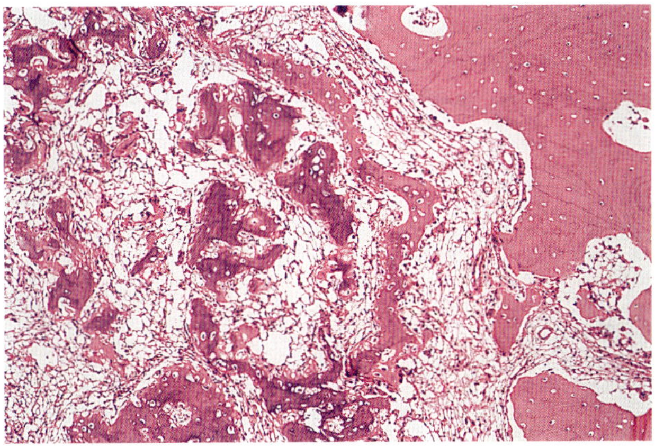

Figure 3-45. Osteoid osteoma. Higher magnification of osteoid osteoma exhibiting osteoid formation in the nidus.

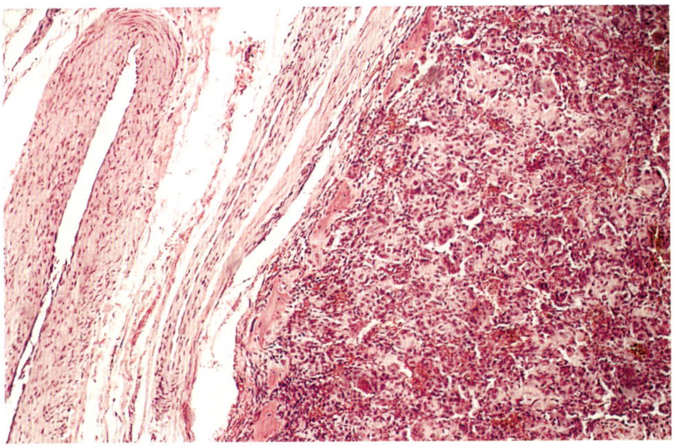

Figure 3-46. Osteoblastoma. Although osteoid formation is readily identified, the lesion is very hemorrhagic and a definite decision regarding the malignant or benign characteristics of the tumor cell cannot be made without help of the margin. A rim of reactive bone with circumscribed growth pattern is an essential feature in the diagnosis of osteoblastoma.

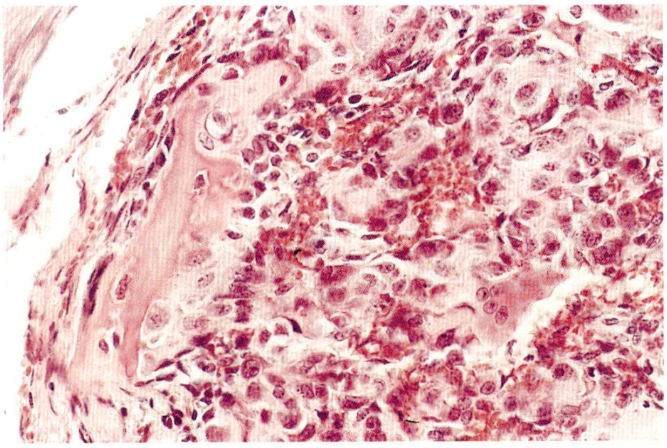

Figure 3-47. Osteoblastoma. Higher magnification of the reactive rim of bone at the edge of an osteoblastoma. Note the extensive hemorrhage within the tumor and the accompanying giant cells.

DIFFERENTIAL DIAGNOSIS, OSTEOID OSTEOMA, OSTEOBLASTOMA AND OSTEOSARCOMA

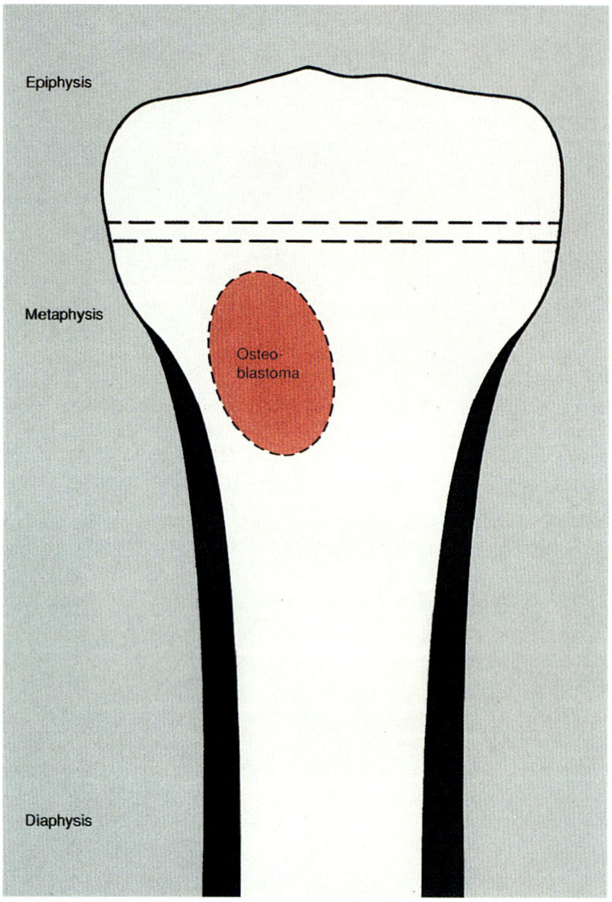

Figure 3-48. Osteoblastoma. Although the osteoblastoma is usually a lesion found in the vertebral column, osteoblastomas may also involve long bones. When they do they are in the same general area as the osteosarcoma, on the metaphyseal side of the growth plate. They are sharply circumscribed lesions, with definable margins. Osteoblastomas may or may not calcify: although immature osteoid is formed by an osteoblastoma, it need not calcify.

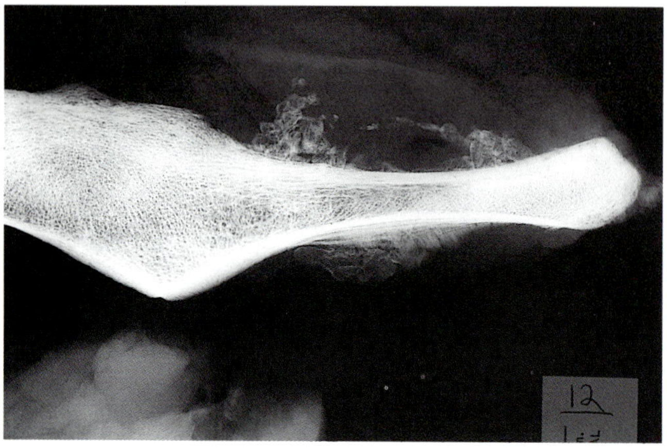

Figure 3-49. X-ray of osteosarcoma of scapula. Note permeative destruction of matrix, permeation through the thin cortical margin, and extensive periosteal reaction, including a laminated and hair-on-end reaction. The tumor extends outside the bone into the adjacent soft tissue and exhibits an irregular calcific pattern in the soft tissue.

plastic cartilage, also *must* have some areas of neoplastic bone formation (Figures 3-58 to 3-61 and 4-45).[14,15]

CAT scan is essential to differentiate juxtacortical osteosarcomas from conventional osteosarcoma extending through the cortex.

Malignant Transformation of Paget's Disease

Paget described malignant transformation in five of his 23 original patients. Since Paget's disease involves the osteoblastic, osteoclastic, and fibroblastic cell lines, tumors that arise in this setting not surprisingly consist of osteosarcomas or osteoblastomas, giant cell tumors, fibrosarcomas, or malignant fibrous histiocytomas.

Several centers have published their experiences with sarcomas arising in Paget's disease.[16–19] All studies agree on the predominance of osteosarcoma and the relative lethality of these secondary tumors, compared wtih primary bone sarcomas arising in a comparable age group. Affected persons often present with increasing pain and a mass. On radiography the preexisting sclerotic Paget's bone is destroyed by the expanding malignant tumor. Less frequently observed but nevertheless a reliable sign is the demonstration of a soft-tissue mass extending outside the cortex, or the presence of a periosteal reaction.

Histologically, the diagnosis of a secondary sarcoma is not difficult since these tumors are anaplastic, high grade lesions. One of the earliest histological changes of sarcomatous degeneration is the reappearance of a cellular spindled stroma in the medullary cavity. In the osteosarcomas, true malignant osteoid production may be scanty and difficult to detect, and therefore the osteoblastic phenotype of the sarcoma may not be present in a small biopsy sample. On the other hand, there is a tendency to misinterpret fibrosarcomas and malignant fibrous histiocytomas as osteosarcomas because of the presence of acellular hyalinized ribbons of collagenous fibrous tissue mimicking osteoid. The distinction may

DIFFERENTIAL DIAGNOSIS OF JUXTACORTICAL LESIONS

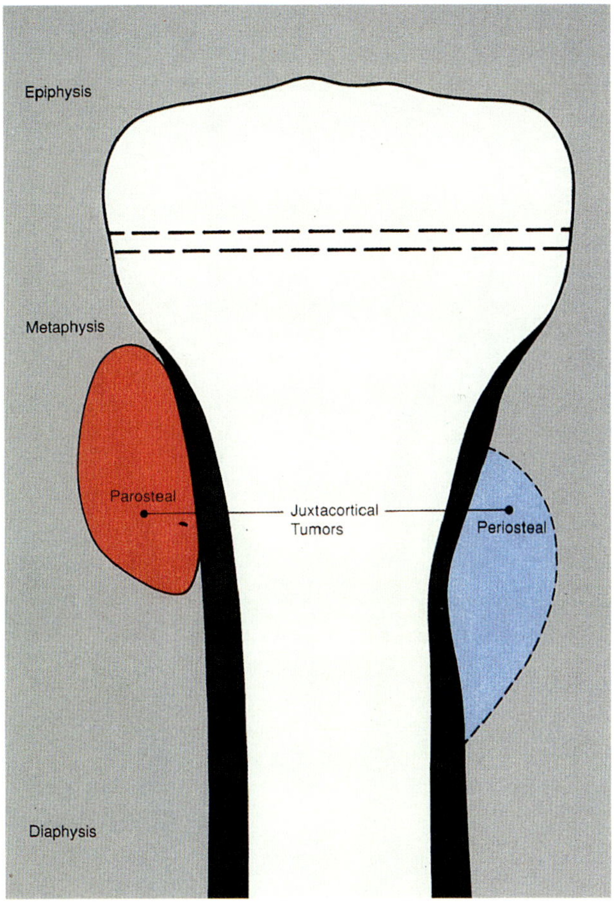

Figure 3-50. Juxtacortical tumors are usually associated with either parosteal or periosteal growth patterns. The parosteal growth pattern is illustrated as superficial to the periosteal membrane and cortex, and is usually a well-differentiated osteosarcoma with slow growth pattern. To differentiate it from a myositis ossificans, the parosteal tumor does not have evidence of peripheral maturation, and the least differentiated portion is at the periphery. The juxtacortical periosteal osteosarcoma is a mixture of bone and cartilage, although the cartilage component may be predominant. The periosteal tumor usually indents the cortical margin, and is usually located somewhat more metaphyseal than the parosteal sarcoma. In addition to the sarcomas there are juxtacortical chondromas, and juxtacortical fibromas. All of these lesions are rare, one must be careful not to confuse a benign juxtacortical cartilage proliferation with a true juxtacortical periosteal osteosarcoma. In addition to the well-differentiated slow-growing tumors, there are also occasional poorly differentiated juxtacortical (parosteal) osteosarcomas, quick to invade the medullary cavity, and bearing the same prognostic features as any other intracortical osteosarcoma.

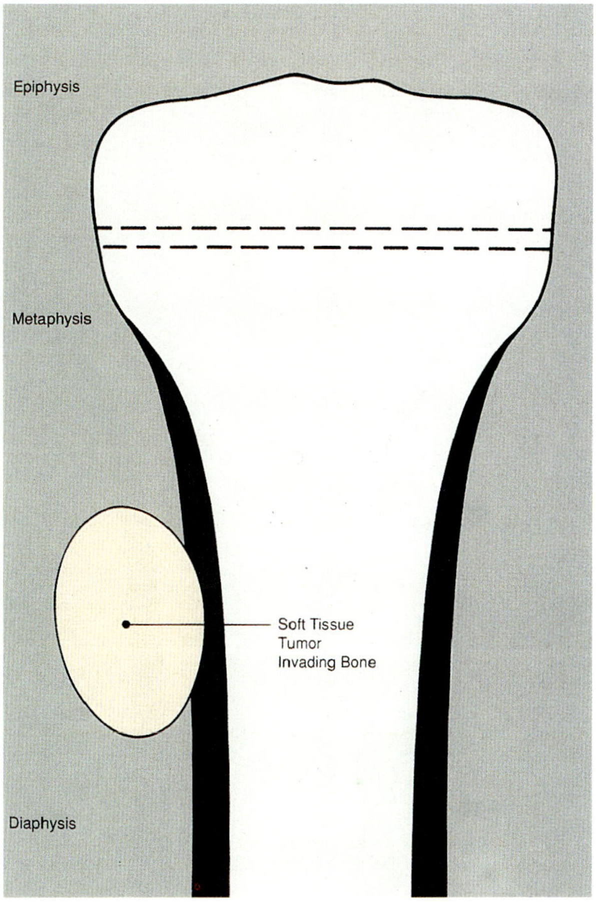

Figure 3-51. Soft tissue tumor invading bone. The rhabdomyosarcomas, fibrosarcomas, synovial sarcomas, and any other type of soft tissue sarcoma may occasionally approach the cortical margin and penetrate through the cortex into the underlying bone structure. At that point it is difficult to determine whether the lesion is a primary tumor of bone extending into soft tissue or vice versa. However a soft tissue tumor does not, as a rule, elicit a periosteal reaction. Instead it indents the cortex; one can usually establish the fact that this indentation is due to the soft tissue mass, which is predominant and extensive outside the bone.

DIFFERENTIAL DIAGNOSIS OF JUXTACORTICAL LESIONS

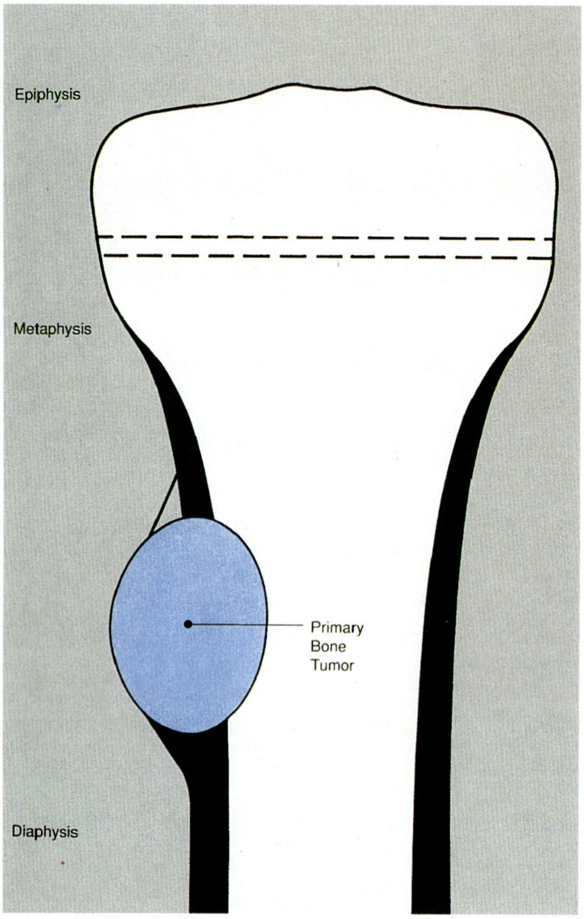

Figure 3-52. Primary tumor of bone emanating from bone and extending into the adjacent soft tissue. This diagram illustrates a primary tumor of bone which forms either a Codman triangle when it is rapid or a buttress when it is slow-growing. The tumor may be any neoplasm, and extension outside the cortical margin is not necessarily an indication of malignancy. However the presence of a Codman triangle would indicate rapid growth associated with malignant tumors, whereas the formation of a buttress would indicate slow and persistent growth, associated with a benign lesion.

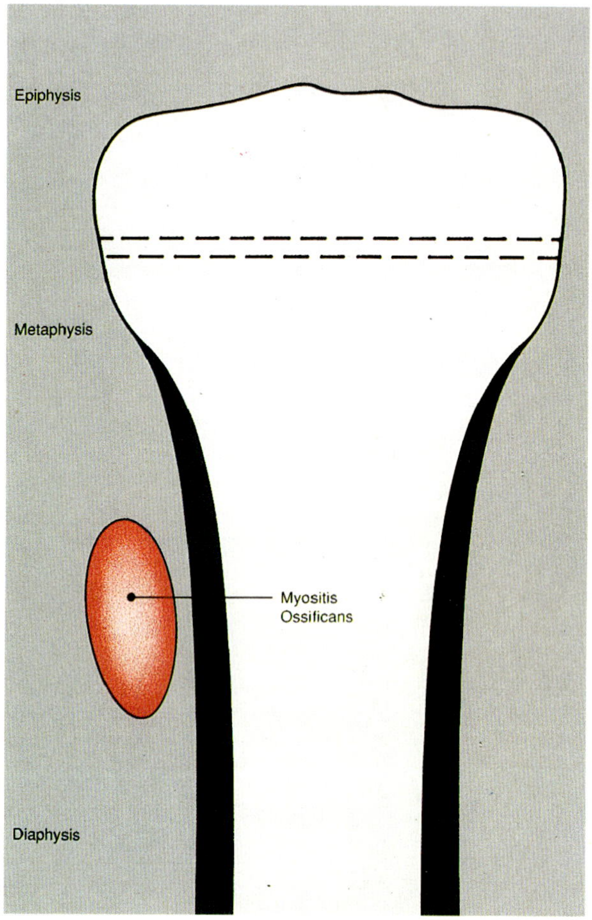

Figure 3-53. Myositis ossificans (heterotopic ossification) (neither myo- nor -itis), represents heterotopic ossification in any mesenchymal component, usually the soft tissue adjacent to the bone. The most important feature of myositis ossificans is the peripheral maturation and sharp delineation against the surrounding soft tissue. This is not clearly visible in the early stages of the proliferation, but as the lesion matures, there should be a sharp delineation against the surrounding tissue, with the most mature features of bone formation at the periphery rather than in the central portion of the lesion. As a rule, myositis ossificans does not attach to bone, but occasionally attachments can be found, and at that time the differential radiographic diagnosis is difficult. However, peripheral maturation and zoning of the histologic material into progressively less mature areas toward the center of the lesion should help to clarify the benign nature of this process, which if left alone will mature into solid bone.

DIFFERENTIAL DIAGNOSIS OF JUXTACORTICAL LESIONS

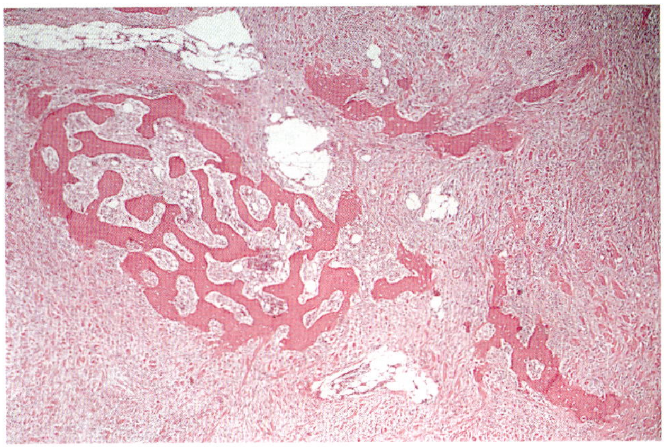

Figure 3-54. Parosteal juxtacortical osteosarcoma. The well-differentiated parosteal osteosarcoma consists of a background of fibrous connective tissue with isolated areas of neoplastic bone formation. The entire picture is one of well-differentiated bone. There is minimal pleomorphism of mitotic activity in the connective tissue elements.

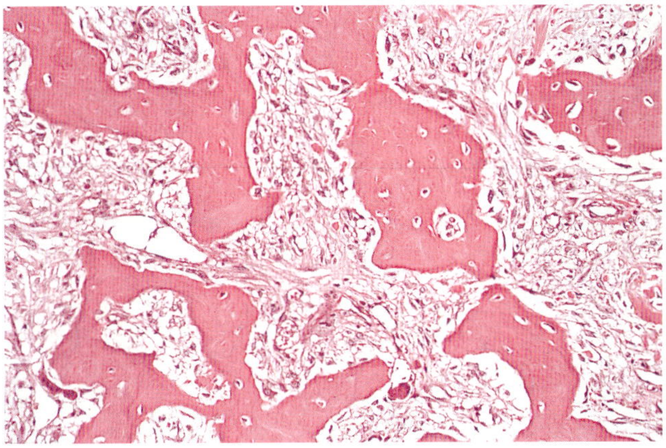

Figure 3-55. Higher magnification of a parosteal osteosarcoma.

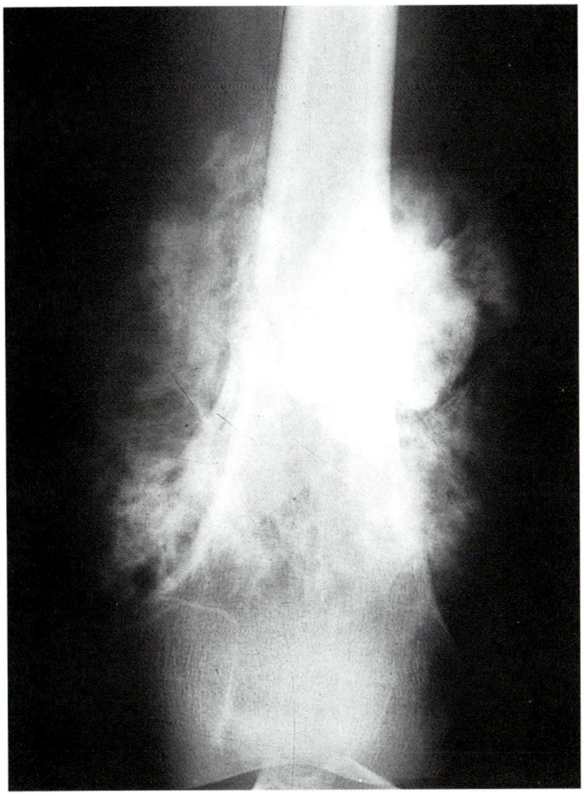

Figure 3-56. A 22-year-old with swelling of lower femur following traumatic episode (falling off horse). The x-rays reveal extensive neoplastic new bone formation, superimposed upon the normal cortical outlines of the lower portion of the femur. CAT scan would confirm that the entire lesion is outside the medullary cavity.

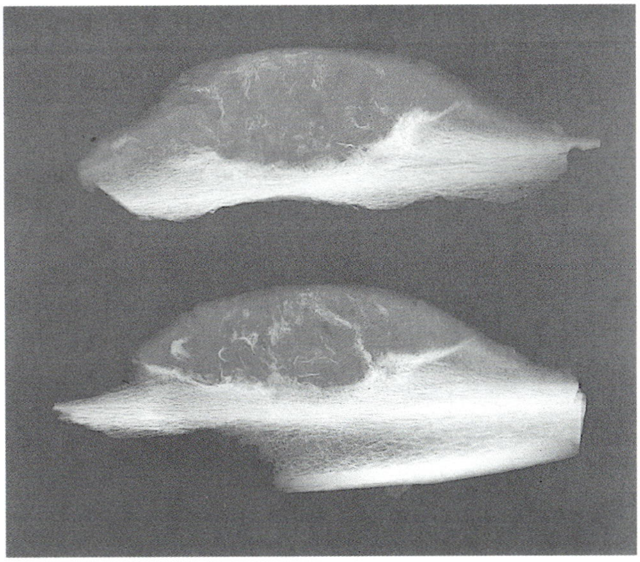

Figure 3-57. Specimen x-ray of periosteal osteosarcoma. Note the predominance of cartilage on the surface of the bone. Despite extensive cartilage formation, a periosteal osteosarcoma must have identifiable fragments of bone formation by the tumor cell.

DIFFERENTIAL DIAGNOSIS OF JUXTACORTICAL LESIONS

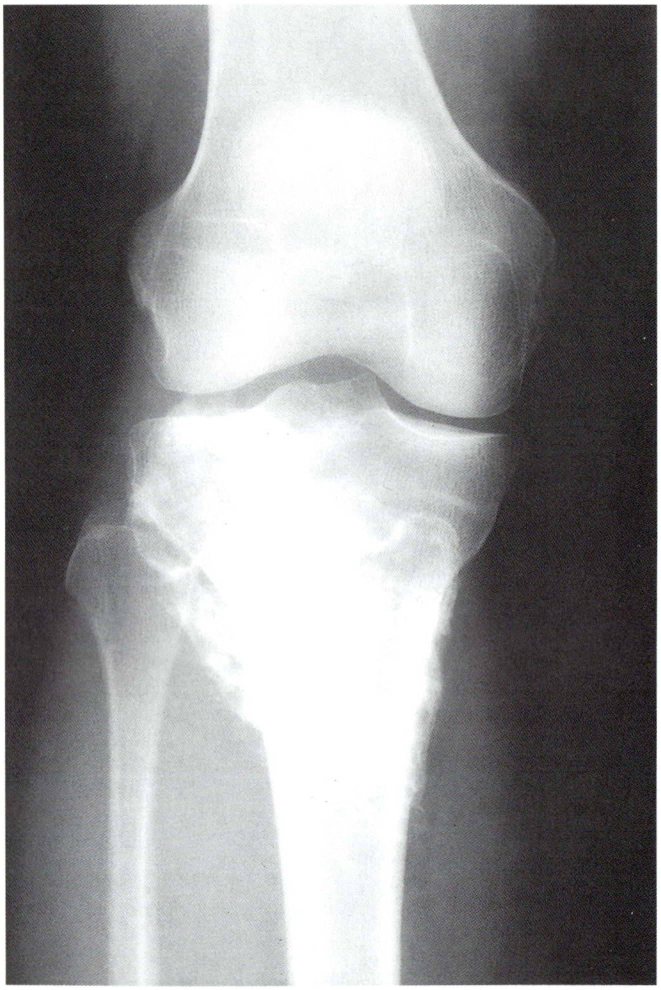

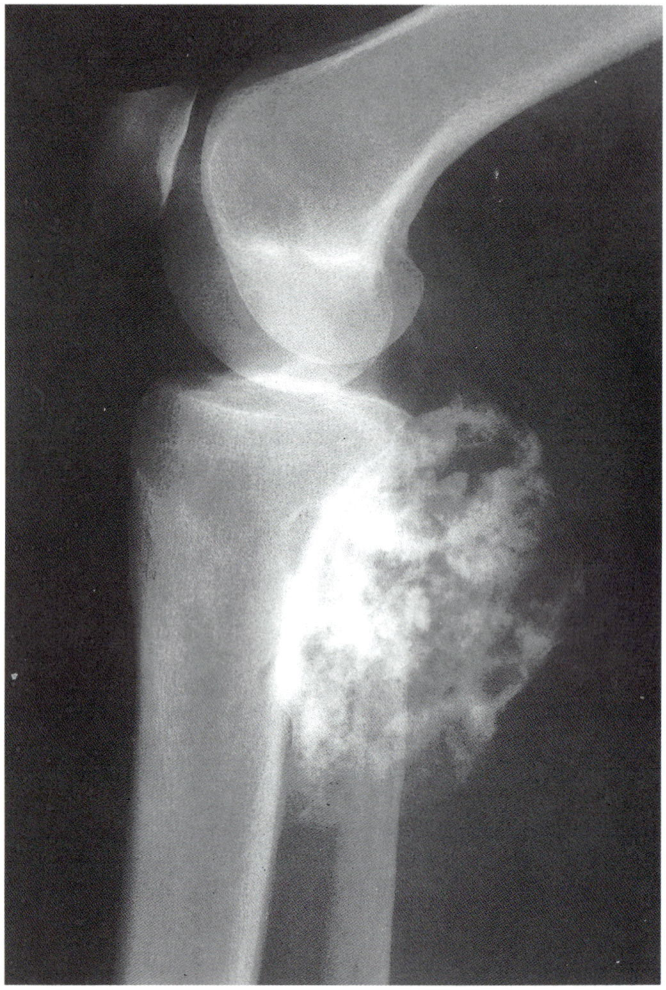

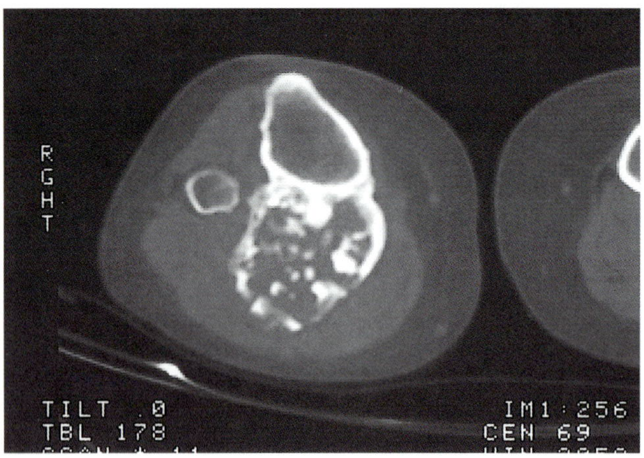

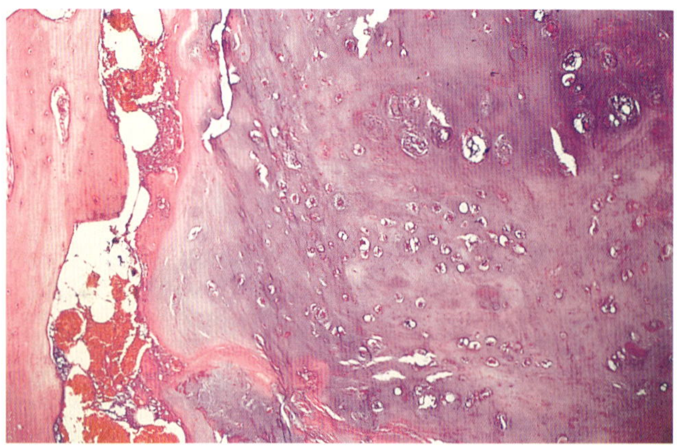

Figures 3-58, 3-59, 3-60, 3-61. Radiographs demonstrating periosteal chondroma. Flocculent calcification adjacent to the proximal tibia is easily demonstrated as an extracortical lesion by CAT scan. The cartilage itself is histologically benign although one must be careful to sample extensively.

not be critical, as all forms of these high grade sarcomas behave similarly, with rapid progression and early metastases (Figures 3-9, 3-10).

Osteoblastoma

Osteoblastoma is a relatively rare lesion producing osteoid with clearly identifiable osteoblasts.[8,20–25] It is often difficult to differentiate from an osteosarcoma, especially the well-differentiated osteoblastoma-like osteosarcoma. The differentiation depends on the following:

1. The osteoblastoma should consist of plump epithelioid osteoblasts with large quantities of cytoplasm and a prominent clear zone within the cytoplasm, identifiable on routine hematoxylin-eosin (H & E) sections.
2. The osteoblastoma should produce geographic osteoid, varying in maturation but producing fairly large masses.
3. The osteoblastoma should grow slowly, and should be clearly defined by a sharp margin, with reactive bone formation. The nature of the more mature bone that is often seen at the periphery of an osteoblastoma is somewhat in doubt; some authors believe this is a normal reactive process on the part of the host, others feel that the osteoblastoma itself is producing this well-demarcated margin. The important issue is that a margin exists, that it is sharply defined, and it corresponds to the geographic margin as seen on the radiograph.
4. An osteoblastoma should *never* produce neoplastic cartilage, or fine lacy osteoid pattern. Neoplastic cartilage or lacy osteoid strongly suggest the presence of osteosarcoma.

Osteoblastomas are often accompanied by numerous giant cells, to the point where the differential diagnosis between an osteoblastoma and a giant cell tumor of bone is considered. The giant cell tumor of bone does not produce large quantities of osteoid. While it may have a large giant cell component, the osteoblastoma is a predominantly osteoid-producing benign neoplasm.

Aneurysmal bone cyst formation secondary to osteoblastoma is not infrequent, and many osteoblastomas exhibit large dilated vascular spaces.

Aggressive Osteoblastoma

Dr. Dorfman has been the foremost proponent of a subclassification, entitled "aggressive osteoblastoma."[26,27] They are characterized by larger, more prominent epithelioid osteoblasts. As in conventional osteoblastoma, there should be no cartilage formation and only minimal quantities of lacy osteoid. Abnormal mitotic figures should not be present. Some of these cases are controversial, and may fall into the well-differentiated osteoblastoma-like osteosarcoma groups. Some observers (Schajowicz) believe the diagnosis of aggressive osteoblastoma should be discouraged; the documented cases of aggressive osteoblastoma turning up with metastatic disease point to the difficulty in establishing the diagnosis. It is a rare lesion; the diagnosis should be made with reservation. Most observers agree that aggressive osteoblastoma is an established entity, to be differentiated from osteosarcoma by the lack of invasive propensity, the lack of the abnormal mitotic figures, and the presence of the large, although benign osteoblasts. The diagnosis should be made with caution.

Osteoid Osteoma

The nidus of an osteoid osteoma is defined as the lytic area in the center of a sclerotic reaction. The nidus should not be larger than 1 cm, although occasional exceptions exist. It is formed by a pattern of proliferation of osteoblasts with osteoid formation, numerous vascular spaces, and numerous giant cells. The osteoid production within the nidus is indistinguishable from osteoid production by an osteoblastoma. Both osteoblastoma and osteoid osteoma exhibit plump benign-appearing osteoblasts without evidence of pleomorphism and certainly no significant mitotic activity. As opposed to the osteoblastoma, the osteoid osteoma will exhibit extensive and excessive bony reaction at the rim of the nidus.[22–24,28,29]

Some individuals consider the osteoid osteoma simply as a small version of the osteoblastoma. This is not an appropriate generalization. Osteoid osteoma is not a neoplasm, it is self-limiting and self-healing if left alone. The osteoblastoma is a progressively growing benign tumor with at least some documented cases of malignant transformation. The biologic potential of both lesions is radically different, therefore they are not variants of a single entity. The location of osteoid osteoma is universal, and while some sites are more favored, there is really no predilection for any given site either within the bone, periosteal, subarticular, metaphyseal, diaphyseal or other.[30] This is in marked contrast to an osteoblastoma which has a predilection for the vertebral column or metaphyseal/diaphyseal portion of the appendicular skeleton. As opposed to osteoblastoma, osteoid osteomas tend to mature at the same rate throughout the lesion. Thus when examining the nidus, any portion of the nidus exhibits the same degree of maturation as any other. It is a subtle hint at the true nature of the process (Figures 3-40 to 3-42; 3-44 to 3-47).

REFERENCES

1. Mirra JM, Picci R, Gold RH: *Bone Tumor, Clinical, Radiologic, and Pathologic Correlations.* Philadelphia, Lea and Febiger, 1989.
2. Meyer WH: Recent developments in genetic mechanisms, assessment, and treatment of osteosarcomas. *Curr Opin Oncol* 3(4):689–693, 1991.
3. Meyer WH, Malawer MM: Osteosarcoma. Clinical features and evolving surgical and chemotherapeutic strategies. *Pediatr Clin North Amer* 38(2):317–348, 1991.
4. Bertoni F, Present D, Bacchini P, et al: The Instituto Rizzoli experience with small cell osteosarcoma. *Cancer* 64(12):2591–2599, 1989.
5. Devaney K, Vinh TN, Sweet DE: Small cell osteosarcoma of bone: an immunohistochemical study with differential diagnostic considerations. *Hum Pathol* 24(11):1211–1225, 1993.
6. Bertoni F, Bacchini P, Fabbri N, et al: Osteosarcoma. Low-grade intraosseous-type osteosarcoma, histologically resembling parosteal osteosarcoma, fibrous dysplasia, and desmoplastic fibroma. *Cancer* 71(2):338–345, 1993.
7. Kurt AM, Unni KK, McLeod RA, et al: Low-grade intraosseous osteosarcoma. *Cancer* 65(6):1418–1428, 1990.
8. Mcleod RA, Dahlin DC, Beabout JW: The spectrum of osteoblastoma. *AJR* 126:321, 1976.
9. Bertoni F, Bacchini P, Donati D, et al: Osteoblastoma-like osteosarcoma. The Rizzoli Institute experience. *Mod Pathol* 6(6):707–716, 1993.
10. Bertoni F, Unni K, McLeod R, et al: Osteosarcoma resembling osteoblastoma. *Cancer* 55:416, 1985.
11. Enneking W, Springfield, D, Gross M: The surgical treatment of periosteal osteosarcoma in long bones. *J Bone Joint Surg* 67A:125–135, 1985.
12. Unni KK, Dahlin DC, Beabout JW: Periosteal osteosarcoma. *Cancer* 37:2476, 1976.
13. Ritts GD, Pritchard DJ, Unni KK, et al: Periosteal osteosarcoma. *Clin Orthop Rel Res* 219:299–307, 1987.
14. Millar BG, Browne RM, Flood TR: Juxtacortical osteosarcoma of the jaws (Review). *Br J Oral Maxillofac Surg* 28(2):73–79, 1990.
15. Raymond AK: Surface osteosarcoma (Review). *Clin Orthop* 270:140–148, 1991.
16. Frassica FJ, Sim FH, Frassica DA, et al: Survival and management considerations in postirradiation osteosarcoma and Paget's osteosarcoma (Review). *Clin Orthop* 270:120–127, 1991.
17. Hadjipavlou A, Lander P, Srolovitz H, et al: Malignant transformation of Paget disease of bone (Review). *Cancer* 70(12):2802–2808, 1992.
18. Healey JH, Buss D: Radiation and pagetic osteogenic sarcomas. *Clin Orthop Relat Res* 270:128–134, 1991.
19. Moore TE, King AR, Kathol MH, et al: Sarcoma in Paget disease of bone: Clinical, radiologic, and pathologic features in 22 cases. *Am J Roentgenol* 156(6):1199–1203, 1991.
20. Boriani S, Capanna R, Donati D, et al: Osteoblastoma of the spine. *Clin Orthop* 278:37–45, 1992.
21. Bettelli G, Tigani D, Picci P: Recurring osteoblastoma initially presenting as a typical osteoid osteoma. Report of two cases. *Skeletal Radiol* 20(1):1–4, 1991.
22. Capanna R, Van Horn J, Ayala A, et al: Osteoid osteoma and osteoblastoma of the talus. *Skel Radiol* 15:360, 1986.
23. Freiberger R, Loitman B, Helpern M, et al: Osteoid osteoma. A report on 80 cases. *AJR* 82:194, 1959.
24. Healey JH, Ghelman B: Osteoid osteoma and osteoblastoma: Current concepts and recent advances. *Clin Orthop Relat Res* 204:76–85, 1986.
25. Kroon HM, Schurmans J: Osteoblastoma: Clinical and radiologic findings in 98 new cases. *Radiology* 175(3):783–790, 1990.
26. Dorfman H, Schiller A: Aggressive osteoblastoma, ilium, with secondary aneurysmal bone cyst. *NEJM* 303:866, 1980.
27. Dorfman H, Weiss S: Borderline osteoblastic tumors: Problems in the differential diagnosis of aggressive osteoblastoma and low grade osteosarcoma. *Semin Diagn Pathol* 1:215, 1984.
28. O'Dell CW Jr, Resnick D, Niwayama G: Osteoid osteoma arising in adjacent bones: Report of a case. *J Can Assoc Radiol* 27:296, 1976.
29. Prabkakar B, Reddy D, Dayananda B, et al: Osteoid osteoma of skull. *J Bone Joint Surg (Br)* 54:146, 1972.
30. Torg JS, Pavlov H, Schwamm HA, et al: Osteoid osteoma: distant, periarticular and intra-articular lesions as a cause of knee pain. *Sports Med* 2:296–304, 1985.

4

Differential Diagnosis of Lesions With Extensive Cartilage

No area in orthopaedic pathology presents as many pitfalls and difficulties to the practicing pathologist as the differential diagnosis of lesions with extensive cartilage. Areas of difficulty include the difference between an enchondroma and a well-differentiated chondrosarcoma; the difference between myxoid chondrosarcoma and lesions with myxoid characteristics, such as chondromyxoid fibroma, chordoma, and myxoid degeneration of neurogenic tumors. A pathologic fracture may often accompany a cartilage neoplasm. Differentiating recent fracture callus with prominent cartilage component from a cartilaginous neoplasm is a problem.

In evaluating a lesion of cartilage, two distinct factors have to be considered: (1) the histologic pattern which establishes the diagnosis, and (2) the biologic potential which attempts to predict the behavior of the neoplasm. One should not confuse the two. Histologic criteria are based on current appearance of the lesion without any further change. These establish the name of the entity, regardless of the patient's age or its location within the bone. Diagnosis as always is based on histologic appearance at the time the lesion is excised.

The biologic potential of a malignant cartilage tumor in the distal appendicular skeleton is low grade. Thus even if there is a chondrosarcoma of any bone distal to the wrist or ankle, experience has shown that those lesions rarely metastasize, and recur locally before distant metastases appear.[1–3] That should not defer the pathologist from calling them what they are: chondrosarcoma with low grade biologic potential.[4] The same lesion in the proximal appendicular or axial skeleton is an ominous affair. In addition to the location within the skeleton, other factors play a role. A child with an open growth plate tends to have greater cellularity in cartilaginous neoplasia than an adult. Thus an enchondroma in a 5-year-old is more cellular than the same enchondroma in a 15- or 20-year-old. Fracture is an additional factor. A pathologic fracture through an enchondroma tends to activate the chondrocytes, and it may therefore exhibit a greater degree of cellularity than the same enchondroma without the pathologic fracture.

Radiologic correlation of these lesions is especially important, since sampling plays such a great role. The margins of an enchondroma should be smooth throughout, sharply circumscribed, and there should be no periosteal reaction. Enchondromas may grow larger, expand the bone, and actually expand into the adjacent soft tissue; that by itself does not make an enchondroma malignant. On the other hand, scalloping of the interior cortical margin of the bone without concurrent thickening of the bone, i.e., scalloping without expansion is a sign of more aggressive activity on the part of the neoplasm and should be viewed with caution. The area of scalloping is the area that should be sampled for biopsy purposes, and the pathologist should attempt to determine where the biopsy took place in postoperative films. In addition to assuring oneself that the most ominous area has been biopsied, one must also assure the surgeon that the material has been adequately sampled, and numerous sections should be prepared of every cartilage neoplasm.[5,6]

ENCHONDROMA VERSUS GRADE I CHONDROSARCOMA

On purely histologic grounds, the enchondroma exhibits uniform nuclei evenly spaced throughout the cartilage matrix, with the nucleus filling less than one-half of the lacunar space. There should be very few double nuclei within one single lacuna, and mitotic figures should be absent. Calcification may be present in any cartilage lesion (Figures 4-1 to 4-8).[7]

As opposed to enchondroma, grade I chondrosarcoma exhibits an increase in absolute number of cells, and diagnosis can be made on the basis of too many cells per unit volume. In addition, there is moderate variation in cell size, shape, and staining, and the cells tend to be plump, fill the lacunar space, with occasional double nuclei or an occasional mitotic figure. Myxoid degeneration of the matrix is an ominous sign. Nevertheless there are times when it is simply impossible to differentiate grade I chondrosarcoma from a cellular enchondroma (Figures 4-9 to 4-12).[8]

Grading of chondrosarcoma correlates well with prognosis, and can be used to manage therapy. Table 4-1 has been adapted from Schajowicz and lists the histologic features that are useful in the grading process. For practical purposes one can simplify the entire grading system as follows: Grade I chondrosarcoma: lesions in which it is difficult to differentiate the tumor from a benign enchondroma; Grade III lesions: basically undifferentiated tumor in which it is difficult to identify the cartilage component of the tumor; Grade II lesions: everything in between.

Aside from the enchondroma, the differential diagnosis must include fracture callus, and osteosarcoma with prominent cartilage component. Osteosarcomas with a large cartilage component do not respond well to pre- or postoperative chemotherapy, and behave much like a poorly differentiated chondrosarcoma. Thus therapy and response to therapy will probably be very similar for either tumor (Figures 4-13 to 4-16).

DEDIFFERENTIATED CHONDROSARCOMA

The "dedifferentiated" chondrosarcoma is a transformation of a low grade chondrosarcoma to a high grade spindle cell tumor, with concurrent worsening of prognosis.[9,10] This dedifferentiated pattern may occur in any low grade chondrosarcoma, and at least in our experience, we have seen sufficient number of enchondromas of the central axial or proximal appendicular skeleton transform into sarcomas with a similar dedifferentiated pattern. The threat of transformation from a benign enchondroma or low grade chondrosarcoma to the dedifferentiated, rapidly growing aggressive lesion requires careful monitoring on the part of the physician taking care of a patient with these entities, and prompt intervention should there be evidence of radiographic or clinical change in a previously quiescent lesion. Histologically the dedifferentiated portion of the chondrosarcoma is difficult to identify as cartilaginous in origin, and only the immediate close proximity and adherence to a clearly definable fragment of neoplastic cartilage identifies dedifferentiated chondrosarcoma[11] (Figures 4-17, 4-18).

CLEAR CELL CHONDROSARCOMA

Clear cell chondrosarcoma is usually located in the epiphysis, with sharp demarcation and geographic boundaries, indicative of slow rate of growth. Radiographically, clear cell chondrosarcoma is difficult to differentiate from chondroblastoma, but usually appears in an older age group.[12,13] The clear cells contain numerous vacuoles which may contain and stain for glycogen. Isolated areas exhibit bona fide cartilage. The tumor may contain areas of calcification, bone spicules,[14] or multinucleated giant cells (Figures 4-19 to 4-22).

Despite innocuous radiographic and histologic appearance, lesions do metastasize. Therefore adequate wide excision rather than curettage is the recommended therapy.

MESENCHYMAL CHONDROSARCOMA

The tumor consists of undifferentiated small cells, mixed with chondroid matrix.[15,16] Many of these cases are in unusual locations (maxilla, mandible, ribs). In addition, from 15 to 35% of these tumors arise in the extraskeletal soft tissues, frequently in meninges, orbit, soft tissues of limbs, neck, chest wall and retroperitoneum. Differential diagnosis includes Ewing's sarcoma, osteosarcoma, and hemangiopericytoma.

The diagnosis of mesenchymal chondrosarcoma depends upon the identification of cytologically malignant foci of cartilage associated with a small cell stroma which may resemble Ewing's sarcoma or hemangioperi-

DIFFERENTIAL DIAGNOSIS OF LESIONS WITH BENIGN-APPEARING CARTILAGE

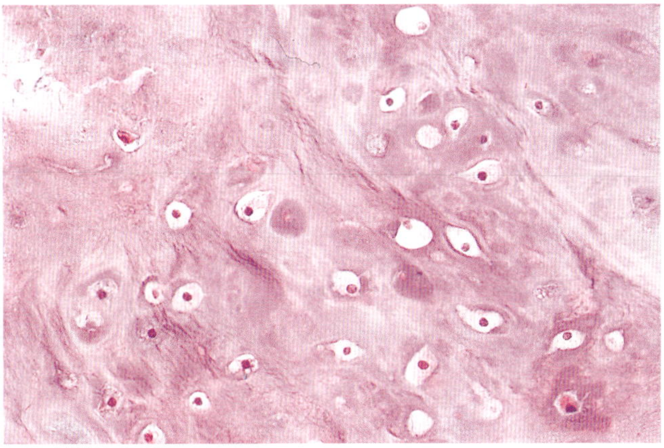

Figure 4-1. Enchondroma. Uniform lacunar spaces, small nuclei filling less than one-third of the lacunar space, uniform matrix formation. Modest cellularity throughout the lesion.

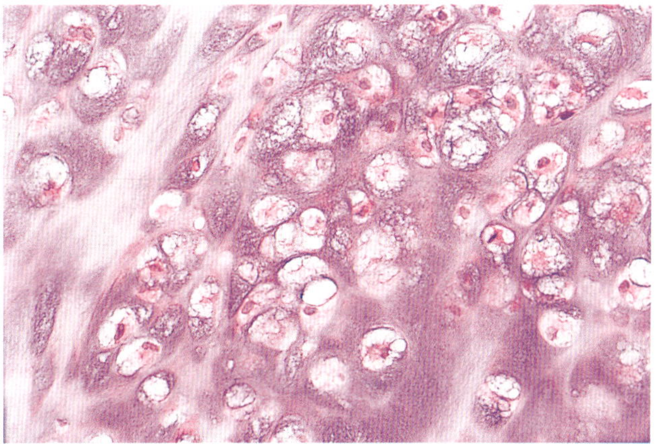

Figure 4-2. Chondrosarcoma, grade I. More prominent nuclei, filling of lacunar spaces, mild pleomorphism. The diagnosis is based strictly on the degree of cellularity, but one assumes that the remainder of the lesion exhibits similar features.

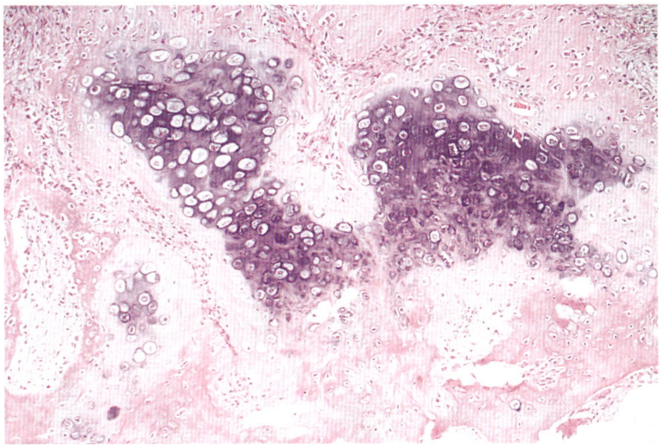

Figure 4-3. Fracture callus. Chondro-osseous bone with cellular cartilaginous component. Note the hypercellularity of the cartilage, and the transition to pink staining osteoid without loss or transition of nuclei.

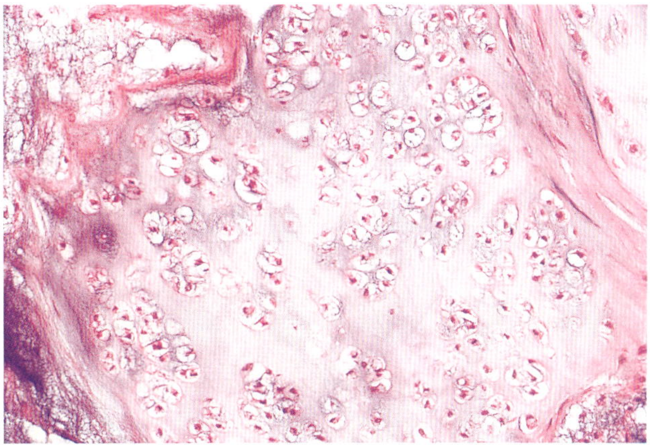

Figure 4-4. Grade I chondrosarcoma with increased cellularity, moderate pleomorphism of the cartilaginous elements.

DIFFERENTIAL DIAGNOSIS OF LESIONS WITH BENIGN-APPEARING CARTILAGE

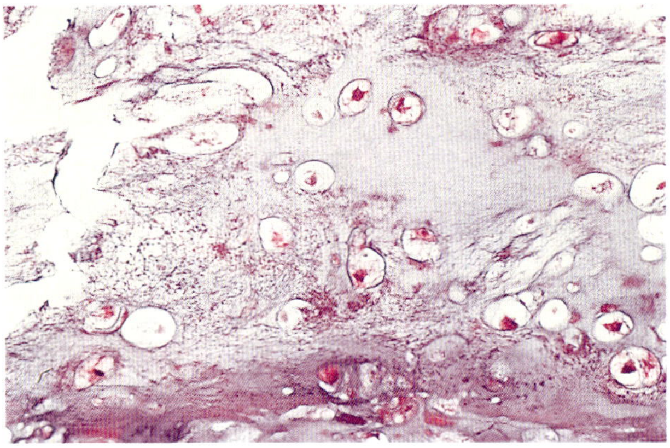

Figure 4-5. Cellular enchondroma with mild atypia. Although the cells are still small, and take up less than one-third of the lacunar space there is mild variation in cell size, shape, and staining. Some myxoid change is present in the matrix.

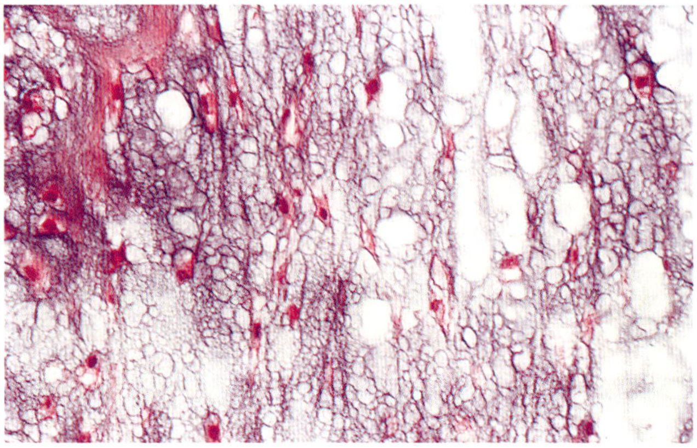

Figure 4-6. Grade I chondrosarcoma. Loss of nuclear space with loss of lacunae and replacement of matrix by myxoid alteration.

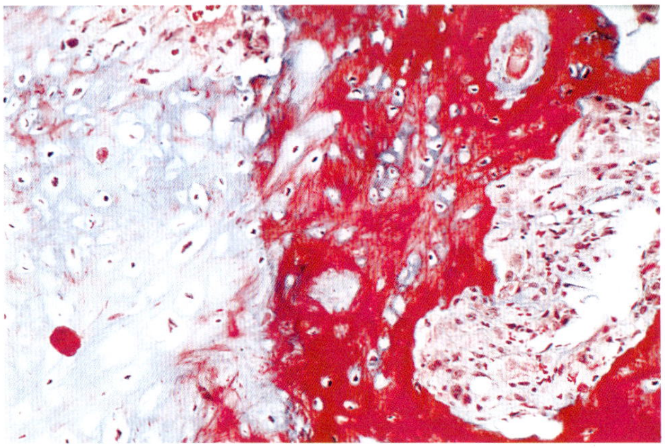

Figure 4-7. Chondro-osseous bone, fracture, Masson trichrome stain. The trichrome stain is useful in demonstrating the transition from cartilaginous to osseous matrix without any change in the nuclear component of the tissue.

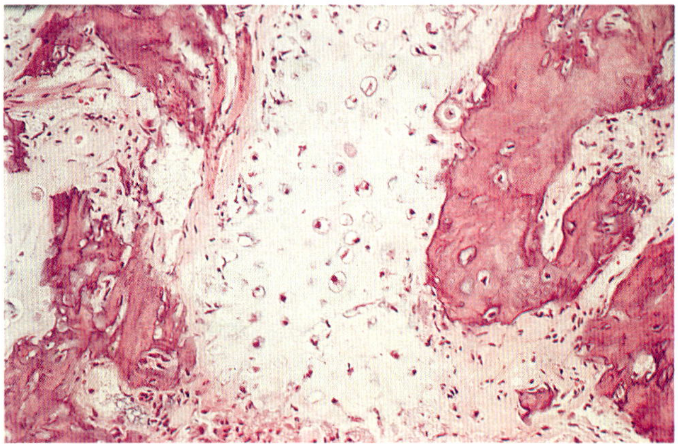

Figure 4-8. Neoplastic cartilage with abutment against adjacent bone fragments. Grade I–II chondrosarcoma.

DIFFERENTIAL DIAGNOSIS OF LESIONS WITH BENIGN-APPEARING CARTILAGE

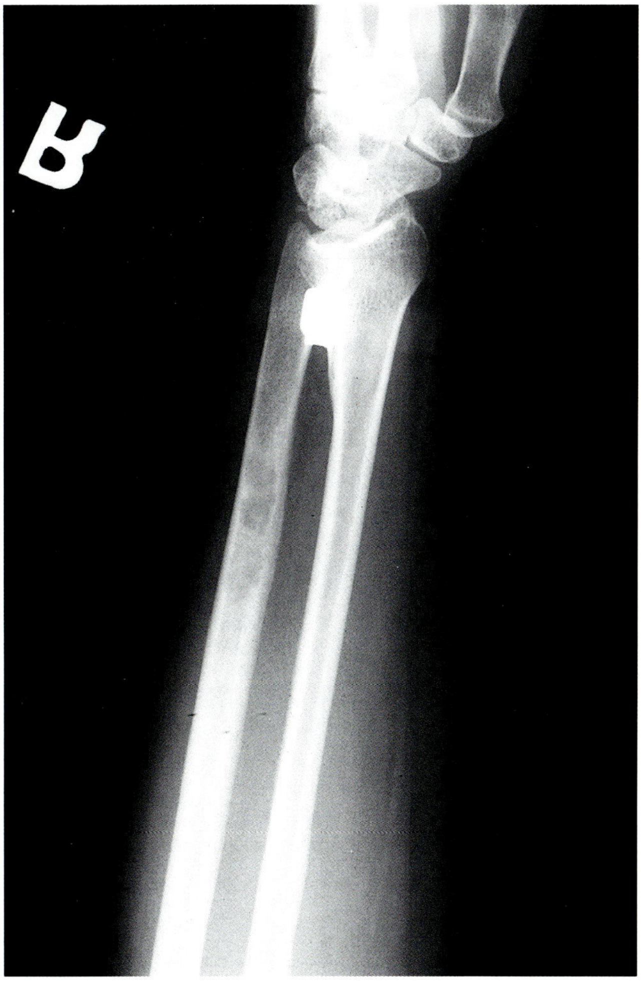

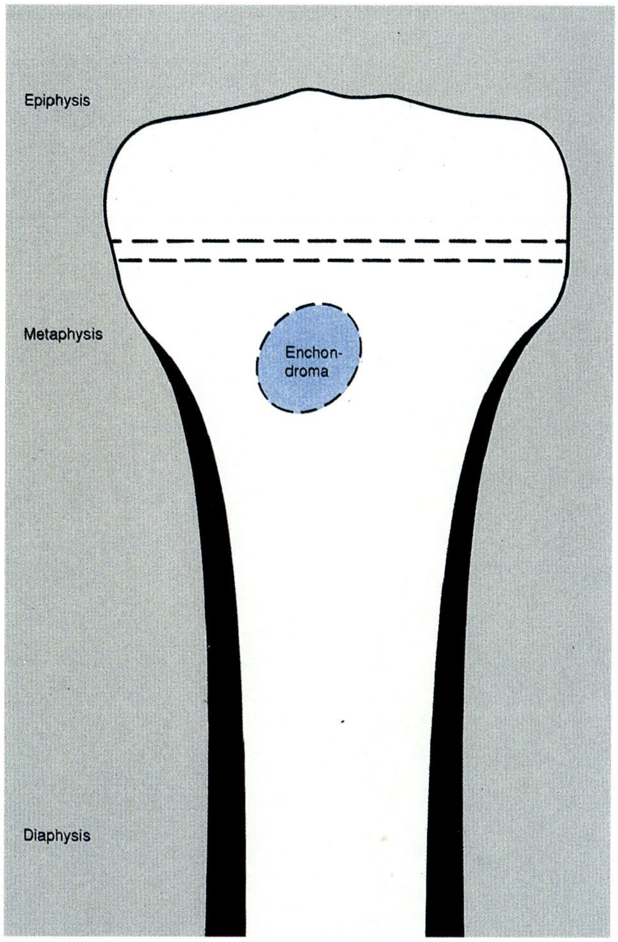

Figures 4-9, 4-10. Enchondroma. The enchondroma is usually a sharply circumscribed defect in bone, lytic, with a reasonable margin of reactive bone confining the lesion to a sharply defined geographic area. Most enchondromas are located in the metaphysis, although some may be found anywhere in the bone, depending upon the age and evolution of the bone at the time of origin of the lesion. Patients with Ollier's disease (multiple enchondromatosis) have enchondromas in the epiphysis, metaphysis, and diaphysis, and many of those lesions are not discernible by simple radiographic analysis.

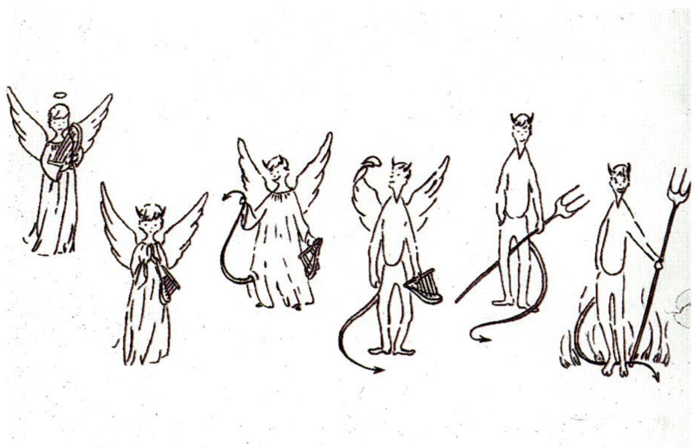

Figure 4-11. At times the difference between enchondroma and grade I chrondrosarcoma is difficult.

DIFFERENTIAL DIAGNOSIS OF LESIONS WITH BENIGN-APPEARING CARTILAGE

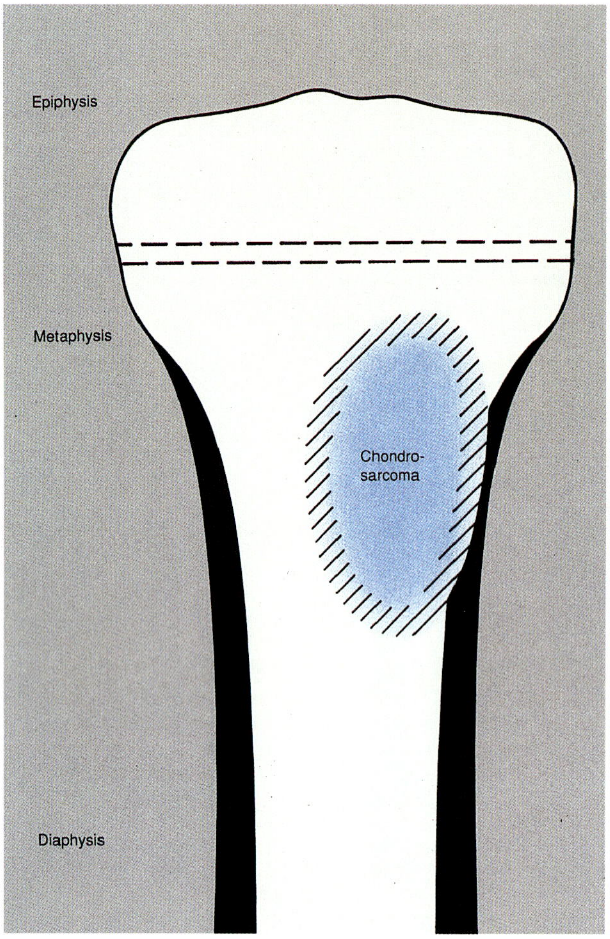

Figure 4-12. Chondrosarcoma. The chondrosarcoma is a malignant tumor, but may have different rates of growth. The margins are usually moth-eaten, but may be permeative. A telltale mark is the encroachment upon the cortical margin on the endosteal side of the cortical margin (scalloping of the cortex). Scalloping is defined as erosion of the internal surface of the cortex without any compensatory reinforcement on the external margin. This indicates aggressive growth and fairly rapid destruction, consistent with a neoplastic malignant process. On the whole, most chondrosarcomas are slower growing than their osteoid counterparts, but one should not be misled by the relatively slow growth and relatively more confined characteristics of the chrondrosarcoma into belittling its malignant potential.

TABLE 4-1. Grading of Chondrosarcomas

Cytologic Pattern	*Low Grade*	*Moderately Malignant*	*Highly Malignant*
Variation of nuclear size	Slight. Moderate number of plump nuclei.	Moderate. Many plump nuclei.	Evident polymorphism. Large number of plump nuclei.
Double nuclei	Low incidence. May be plump.	Frequent. Plump double nuclei.	Numerous
Multinucleated atypical giant cells	Absent	Absent or rare	Occasional–frequent
Calcification	Frequent, conspicuous	Occasional	Absent or scarce

Adapted from Schajowicz F: *Tumors and Tumorlike Lesion of Bone. Pathology, Radiology, and Treatment.* New York: Springer-Verlag, 1994.

DIFFERENTIAL DIAGNOSIS OF CARTILAGE TUMORS

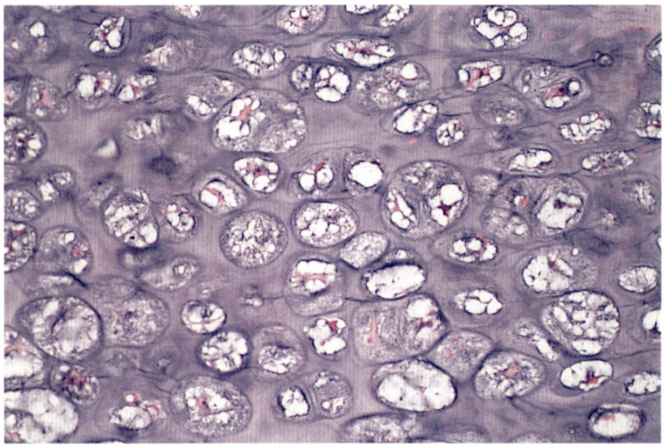

Figure 4-13. Grade I chondrosarcoma. Crowding of cellular material, filling of the lacunar space, extensive myxoid change within the lacuna.

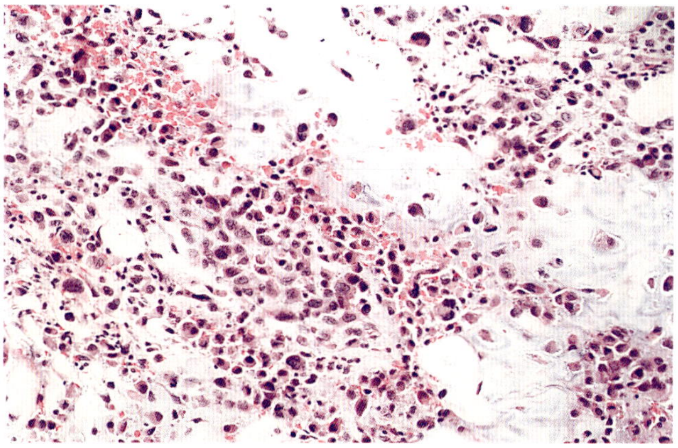

Figure 4-14. Chondrosarcoma, grade III. Clearly identifiable cartilage is present. The cellular elements of the tumor exhibit moderate pleomorphism and irregular chromatin pattern. Although clearly identifiable cartilage is being produced by portions of the tumor, the cellular components lack any further differentiation, classifying the lesion as a grade III chondrosarcoma.

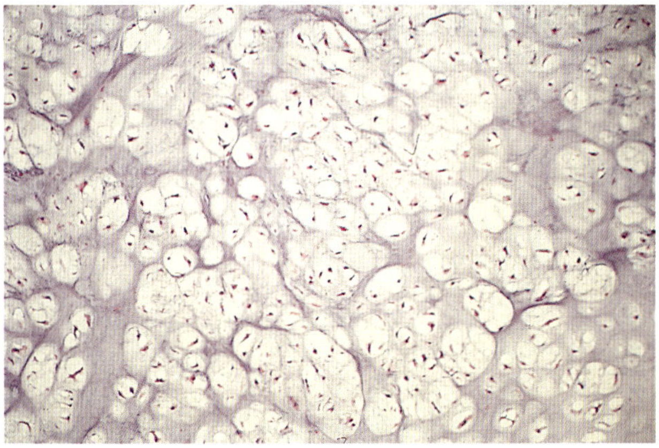

Figure 4-15. Grade I chrondrosarcoma. Even though nuclear material is small, lacunar spaces are large, and there is no evidence of mitotic activity, the degree of cellularity is excessive and indicates a chondrosarcoma.

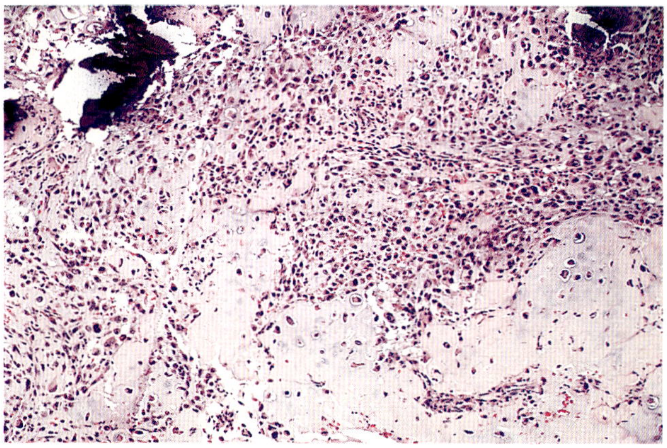

Figure 4-16. Grade III chondrosarcoma. While there are areas of cartilage differentiation, the cellular component of the tumor is extremely pleomorphic with marked hyperchromatism of nuclei, variation in size, shape, and staining. Focal areas of calcification are noted.

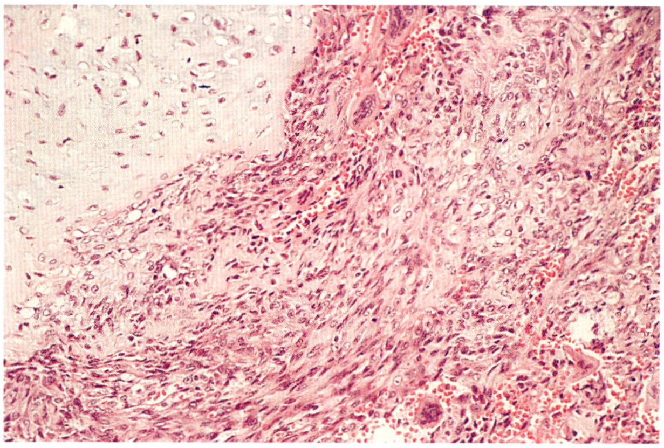

Figure 4-17. Dedifferentiated chondrosarcoma. Note the malignant fibrous histiocytoma (MFH)–like pattern of the tumor, adjacent to a grade I chondrosarcoma.

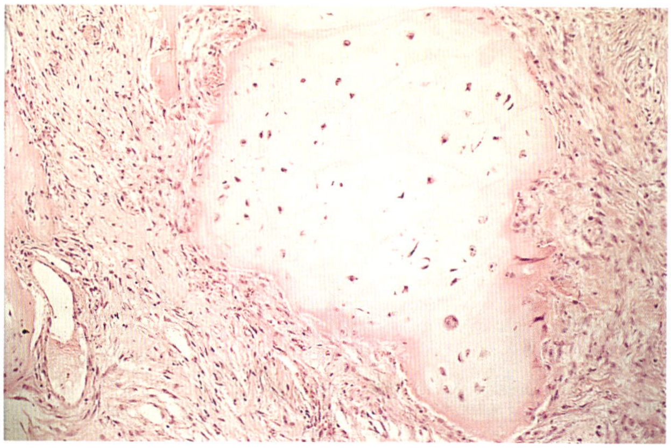

Figure 4-18. Dedifferentiated chondrosarcoma. Benign cartilage proliferation, adjacent to malignant transformation to MFH-like pattern.

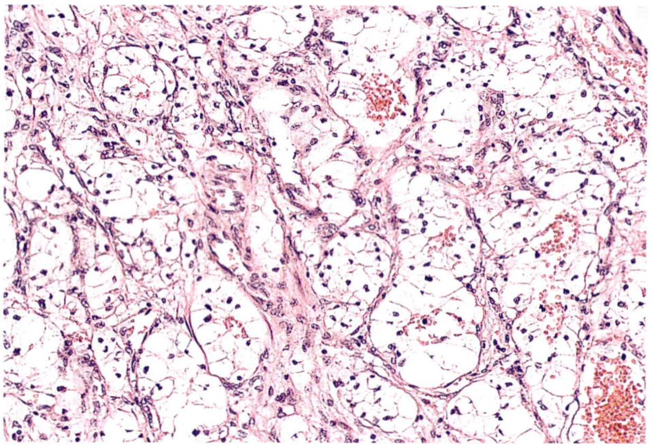

Figure 4-19. Primary renal cell carcinoma in the kidney demonstrating the clear cell pattern which can be seen in the spindled metastatic tumor.

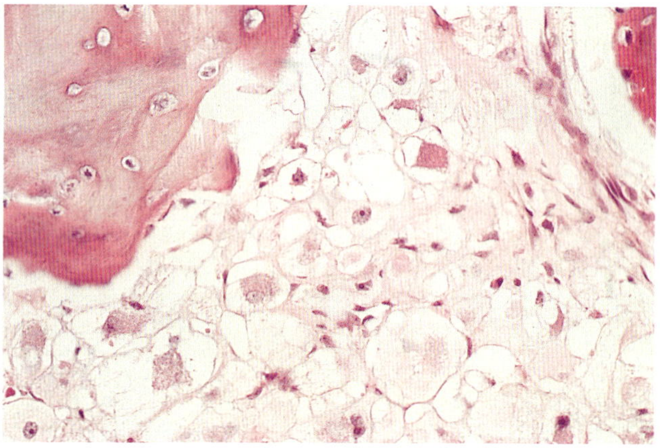

Figure 4-20. Clear cell chondrosarcoma with readily identifiable clear cells adjacent to bony trabeculae.

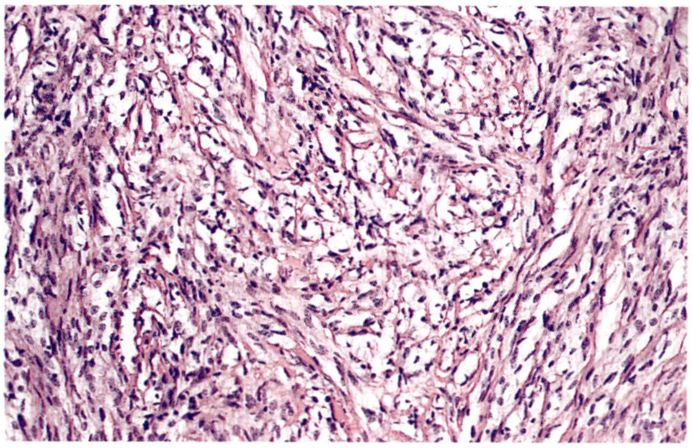

Figure 4-21. Same tumor as in Figure 4-19. Note the clear cell pattern prevalent in the midst of what appear to be spindled cells but in reality are spindled epidermal cancer cells. Again the clear cells may be confused with a histiocytic tumor, and misinterpreted as xanthoma cells. Immunohistochemistry will readily resolve the issue.

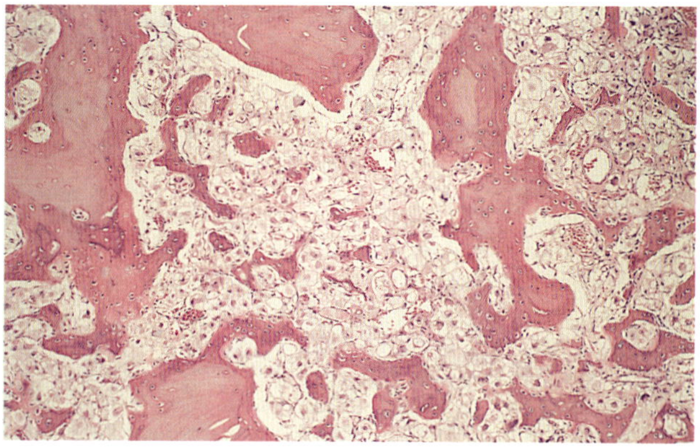

Figure 4-22. Clear cell chondrosarcoma. The cartilage component of this neoplasm infiltrates the trabecular bone pattern just like in any other chondrosarcoma. The bone is not formed by the tumor, but rather a reactive process.

cytoma. The two components are always closely admixed. (See the discussion of differential diagnosis of round cell tumors in chapter 7, p 104, Figures 7-5, 7-6).

CHONDROMYXOID FIBROMA

The chondromyxoid fibroma is composed of spindled cells with the formation of pink staining collagen fibers connecting the separate spindle-shaped nuclei. They are set in a chondroid, myxoid matrix, but usually there is little if any clearly identifiable cartilage in these lesions. Occasional zones of hypercellularity accompany this fibrous connective tissue and giant cells are often present. The differential diagnosis includes myxoid chondrosarcoma.[17]

The radiographic appearance of a chondromyxoid fibroma is always that of a sharply circumscribed lytic defect in bone, most commonly in the lower extremity; metaphyseal, eccentric, with sharply circumscribed margins. The radiographic appearance is identical to that of a nonossifying fibroma of bone (Figures 4-23 to 4-29).

DIFFERENTIAL DIAGNOSIS OF MYXOID LESIONS

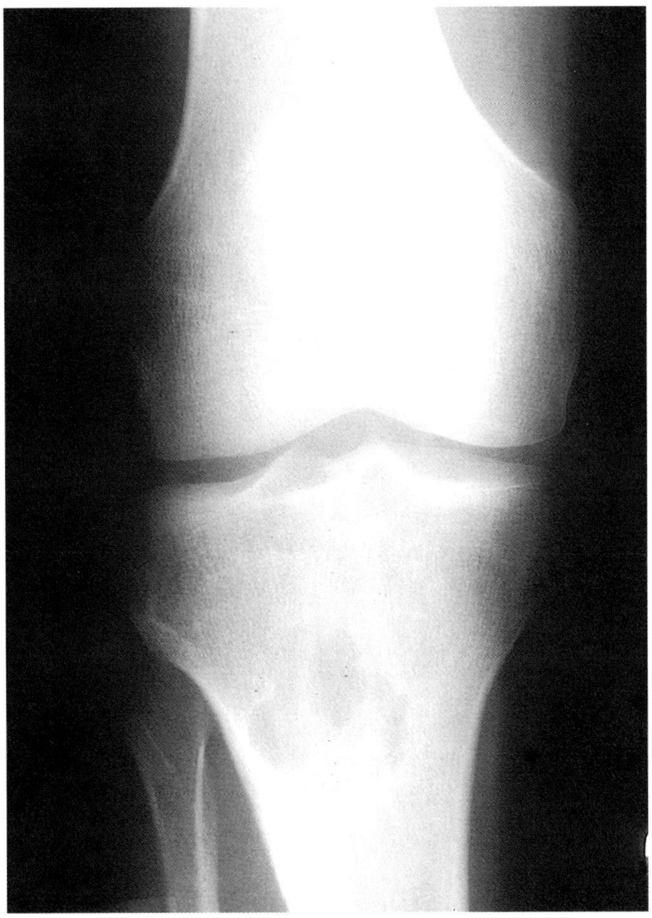

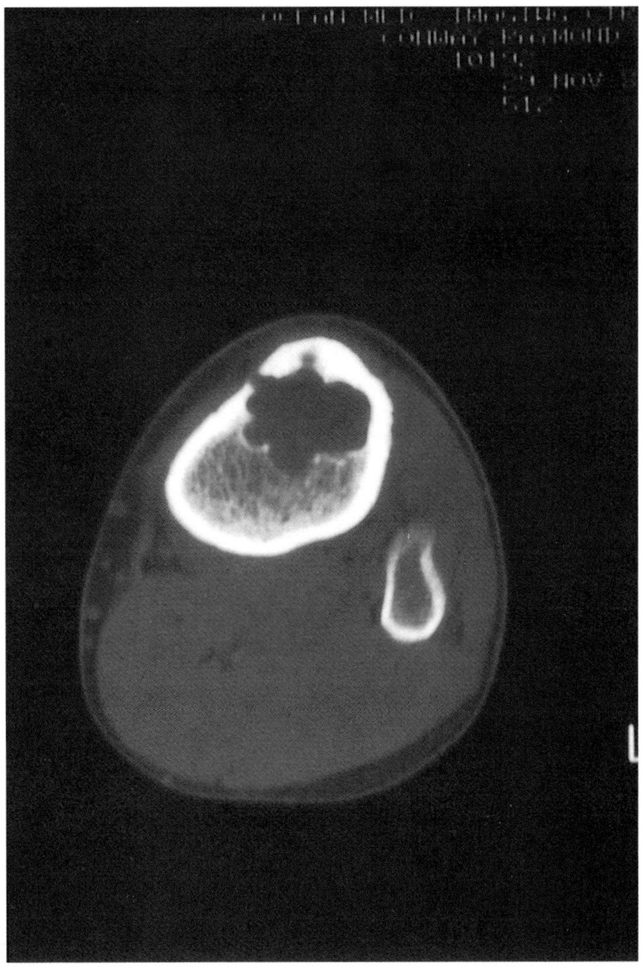

Figures 4-23, 4-24. Chondromyxoid fibroma. The radiograph exhibits a sharply circumscribed eccentric metaphyseal lesion, with no evidence of matrix calcification and no periosteal reaction. The CAT scan confirms the impression, although there is some evidence of endosteal scalloping.

DIFFERENTIAL DIAGNOSIS OF MYXOID LESIONS

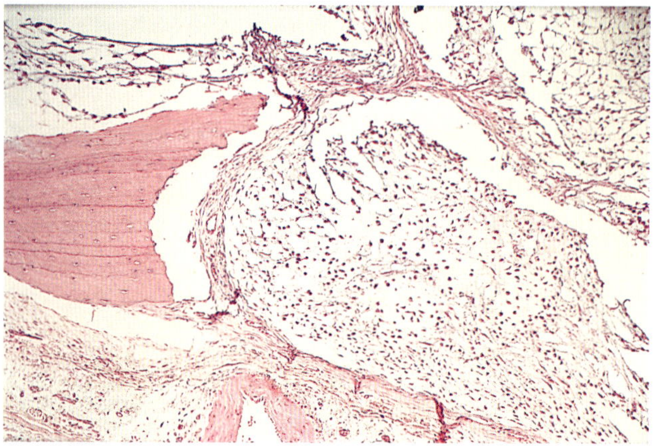

Figure 4-26. Myxoid chondrosarcoma. The cells exhibit loss of lacunar space, with increased cellularity, and penetration with erosion of trabecular bone, indicating an aggressive growth pattern.

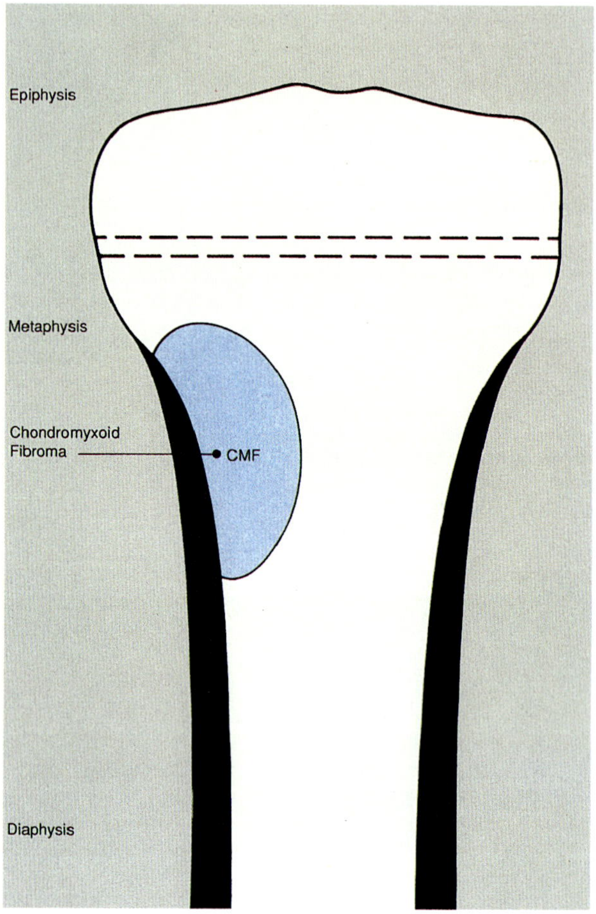

Figure 4-25. Radiographic manifestations, chondromyxoid fibroma. The chondromyxoid fibroma is always a metaphyseal lesion, located eccentrically, with a sharply defined rim of reactive bone at the edge of the lesion. It does not elicit a periosteal reaction, and should not have any visible radiographic calcification. Chondromyxoid fibromas can enlarge, especially in the smaller bones, and become all-pervasive. Most chondromyxoid fibromas are smaller, sharply circumscribed, and radiographically indistinguishable from the nonossifying fibroma of bone.

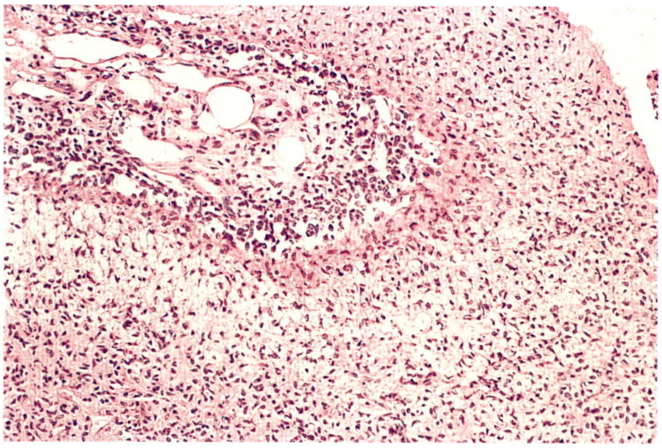

Figure 4-27. Chondromyxoid fibroma. The tumor may be quite cellular, with focal areas of increased cellularity associated with giant cells; there is usually no pleomorphism, no mitotic activity, and although the lesion may at times extend outside the bone, this is not a malignant tumor.

DIFFERENTIAL DIAGNOSIS OF MYXOID LESIONS

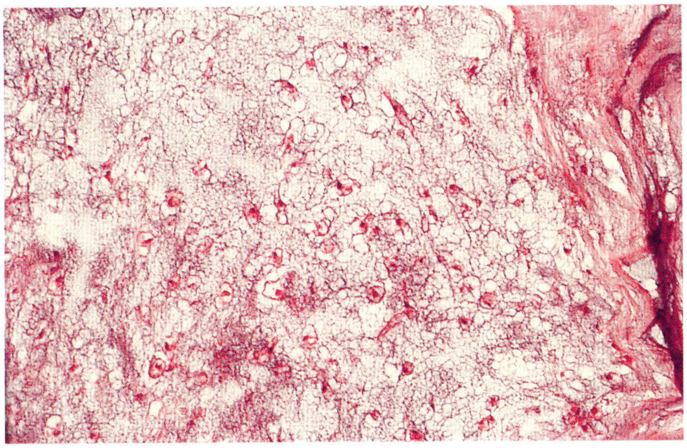

Figure 4-28. Myxoid chondrosarcoma. The sarcoma is characterized by the secretion of extensive myxoid material with only isolated cellular elements in the midst of the myxomatous area. Despite the hypocellularity of the infiltrate, the myxoid component indicates an aggressive pattern of growth, readily penetrating through trabecular and soft tissue planes. The individual nuclei do not have any collagen fiber connection.

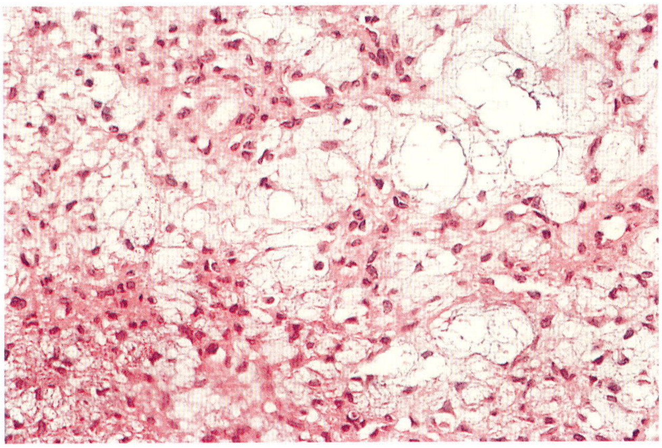

Figure 4-29. Chondromyxoid fibroma. As opposed to a myxoid chondrosarcoma, the chondromyxoid fibroma always has a bridge of collagen fibers extending from one cell to another, sometimes bridging areas of myxoid material.

CHORDOMA

The chordoma is a neoplasm arising from residual notochordal tissue, and therefore restricted to the spinal column. These are malignant tumors, slow growing, but capable of metastatic spread. The relentless but slow growth of the tumor is responsible for the destruction of bone, adjacent soft tissue, or intervertebral disc. In the sacrum these tumors may reach fairly large size before clinical symptoms appear; in the base of the skull or upper cervical vertebral destruction of bone and associated tissues leads to rapid development of symptomatology, usually with fatal consequences.

The histologic hallmarks of the lesion are the production of a physaliphorous cell. This is the classic bubble cell, which consists of a single nucleus with multiple small bubbles arranged in a ring around the nucleus. While these classical features may be present, chordomas may also have simply a sheet-like growth pattern and may resemble epithelioid or signet ring tumors. On the whole, the nuclear structure of these cells is fairly uniform, and mitotic figures are rare. Chordomas may exhibit chondroid differentiation, especially in the more cervical chordomas (Figures 4-30 to 4-33).[18]

The differential diagnosis must include a chondrosarcoma arising in the spine, metastatic adenocarcinoma, and soft tissue tumors, especially liposarcoma. Immunohistochemical analysis with reveal cytokeratin positivity, which would effectively eliminate some of the soft tissue sarcomas and most cases of chondrosarcoma.

CHONDROBLASTOMA (CODMAN TUMOR)

The chondroblast arises in the epiphysis, and is probably the progenitor cell of the numerous cartilage cells which supply the growth plate. It is therefore not surprising that a chondroblastoma is an epiphyseal tumor.

The radiographic presentation of a chondroblastoma is fairly distinctive; a sharply circumscribed lytic defect located predominantly in the epiphysis, with occasional speckled calcification. The tumor is usually confined to the bone, without evidence of periosteal reaction or extension into the adjacent soft tissue, but on occasion an aggressive chondroblastoma may extend into soft tissue. Aneurysmal cyst formation is common.

The histology of the chondroblastoma is varied. Numerous sheets of chondroblasts are identifiable, and these cells are usually sharply circumscribed with very distinctive cellular margins. These margins lead to a description of the lesion as a "bird's-eye view of paving stones." In addition to the polyhedral cellular component, there are usually foci of stippled calcification, fragments of more mature cartilage formation, and numerous giant cells, to the point where the lesion may actually be confused with a giant cell tumor of bone. The characteristic calcification of the lesion has been

DIFFERENTIAL DIAGNOSIS OF MYXOID LESIONS

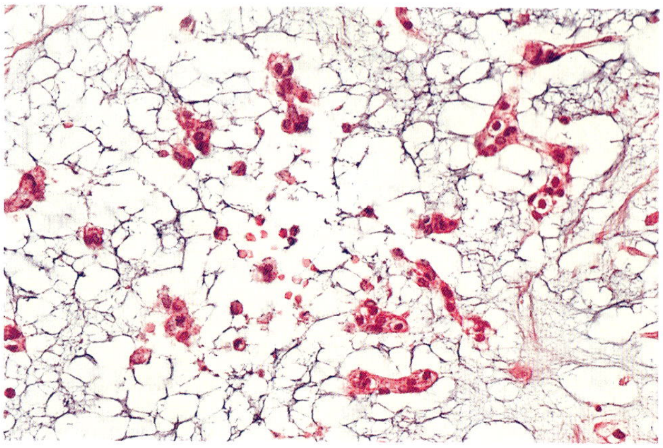

Figure 4-30. Chordoma. Epithelioid-like nests set in myxoid stroma. Note the similarity to the collagen pattern in chondromyxoid fibroma. On this photograph it is difficult to differentiate a chordoma from chondromyxoid fibroma on purely histologic grounds.

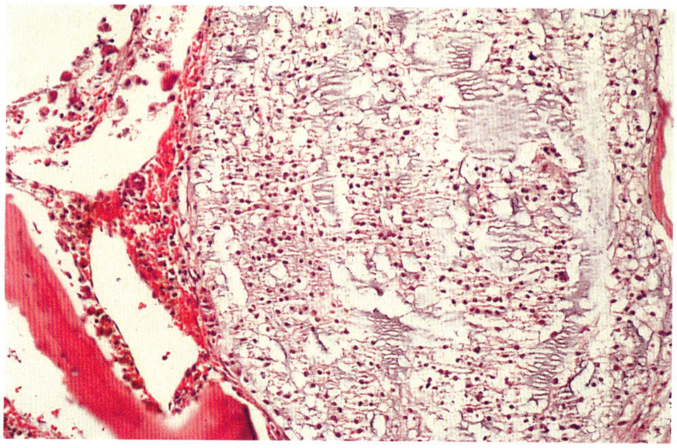

Figure 4-31. Chordoma. The lesion has chondroid characteristics, but is essentially an epithelioid neoplasm which may exhibit immunoreactivity to S100 and keratin. The cells are isolated, without lacunar spaces. Bubbles are present adjacent to the cellular material, corresponding to the physaliphorous differentiation.

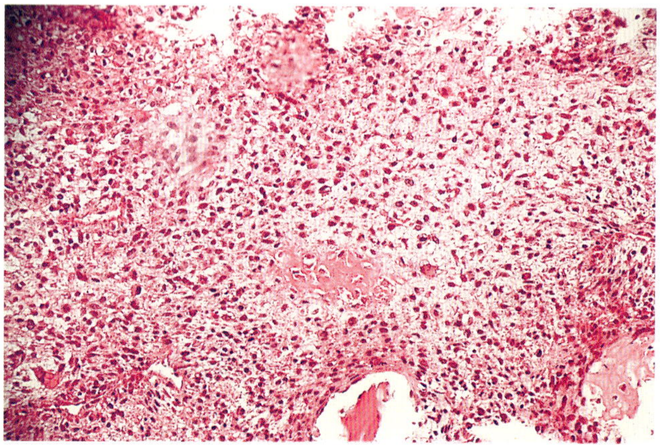

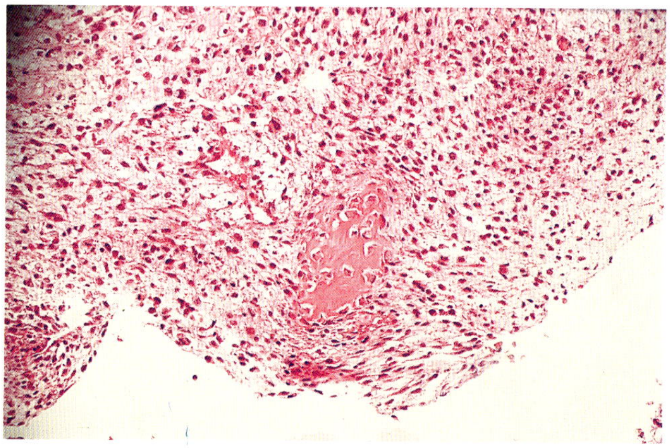

Figures 4-32, 4-33. Chondromyxoid-like osteosarcoma. The lesion exhibits a cellular infiltrate with a myxoid component, similar to the usual chondromyxoid fibroma. However, collagen fibers do not connect cellular elements and focal neoplastic osteoid formation is noted and diagnostic.

classified as "chicken-wire" but more flocculent calcification and actual transformation to bone is also present in numerous lesions.[19,20]

The differential diagnosis includes round cell tumors when one is dealing with the polyhedral cells without paying attention to the cartilage differentiation; a giant cell tumor of bone may be confused with a Codman tumor but one should remember that the giant cell tumor is predominantly metaphyseal, extending into the epiphysis, whereas a chondroblastoma is predominantly epiphyseal and may extend into the metaphysis. Chondroblastomas form cartilage; giant cell tumors of bone may form minute amounts of osteoid. From a radiographic viewpoint the differential diagnosis includes the clear cell chondrosarcoma, which is usually an epiphyseal lesion (Figures 4-34 to 4-39).

CHONDROBLASTOMA

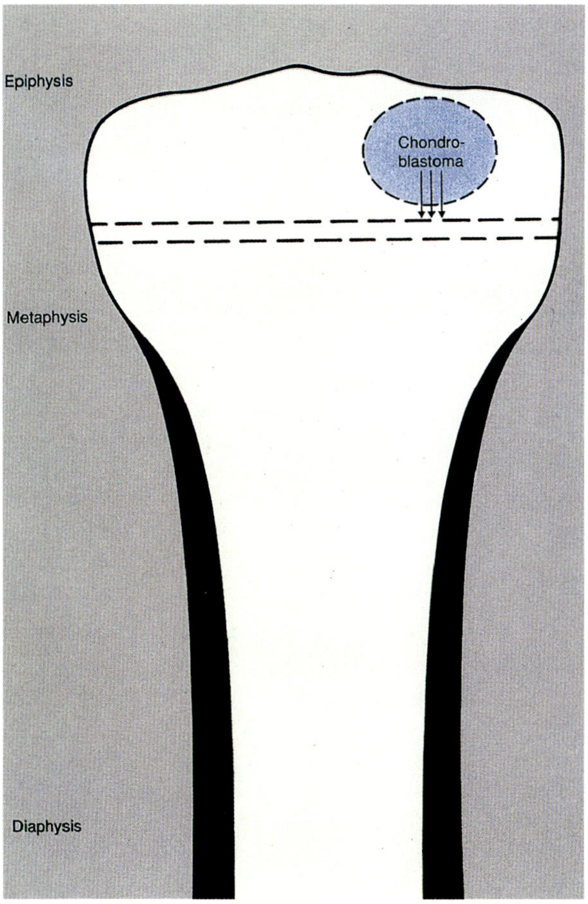

Figure 4-34. Radiographic manifestations of the chondroblastoma. The chondroblastoma is always an epiphyseal (or apophyseal) lesion which extends into the metaphysis only after the growth plate fuses. Chondroblastomas are not present in areas where there is no growth plate. The lesions are sharply circumscribed, lytic, although focal calcification may become visible. Although they may extend into the adjacent soft tissue and have aggressive characteristics, the chondroblastoma is basically a benign tumor, amenable to simple intralesional excision, i.e., curettage.

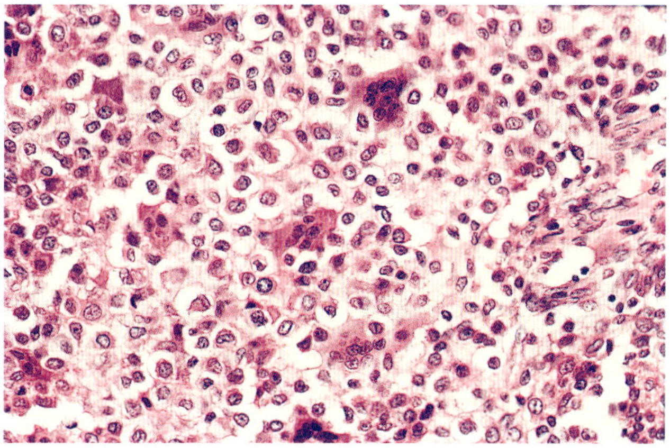

Figure 4-35. Chondroblastoma, numerous giant cells, and identifiable chondroblasts with distinct cell boundaries.

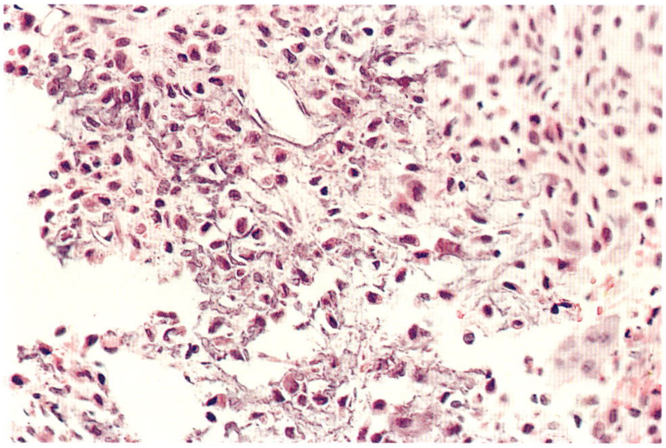

Figure 4-36. Chondroblastoma. "Chicken-wire" classification of chondroblastoma.

CHONDROBLASTOMA

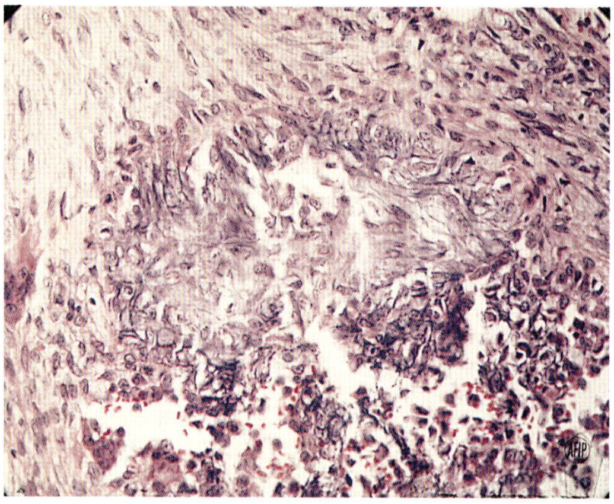

Figure 4-37. Focal calcification pattern seen in chondroblastomas. This calcification pattern is simple calcification by matrix secretion of the neoplastic cells, i.e., an extension of the chicken-wire calcification pattern.

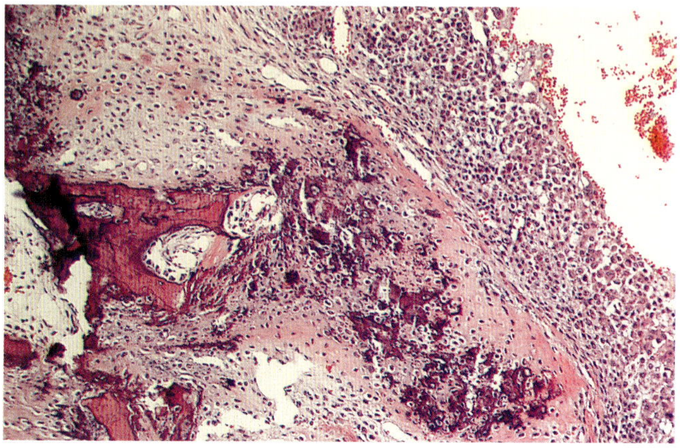

Figure 4-38. Chondroblastoma with calcification and secondary bone formation in association with aneurysmal bone cyst. This chondroblastoma arose in the apophysis of the calcaneus. On the right-hand side of the photograph the typical chondroblast "pavement stone" pattern is identifiable with scattered giant cells. Adjacent to this pattern on one side is the hemorrhagic cyst with numerous red blood cells; on the other side are foci of calcification with pink staining transformation of the matrix. In addition to this calcification pattern there is actual bone formation. Bone formation may result in any tissue that has been calcified. Thus arteriosclerotic vessels, calcified mitral values, thyroid calcification may all proceed to bone formation, and the same applies for calcification in a chondroblastoma.

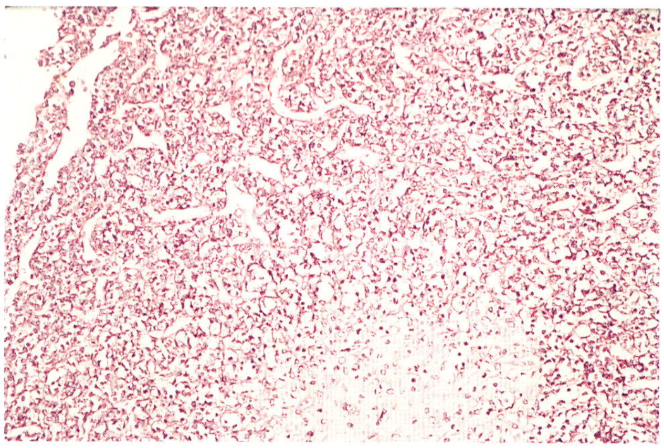

Figure 4-39. Mesenchymal chondrosarcoma. A predominant small cell pattern with only isolated foci of cartilage formation. The small cell pattern by itself could easily be confused with metastatic round cell tumor or even lymphoma.

OSTEOCHONDROMA

The osteochondroma consists of perichondrial proliferation of cartilage with transformation to bone. The lesions may be single or multiple, and may be pedunculated or sessile.[17]

The usual lesion is located on a bony stalk. The pedunculated lesion points in the direction of muscle pull. A sessile lesion is usually located in an area where there is no muscle insertion. Central axial osteochondromas may reach enormous size.

The histology exhibits perichondrium with formation of cartilage, and transformation to bone, mimicking a normal growth plate. The important features establishing the diagnosis include the formation of primary trabeculae with an acellular cartilage core surrounded by osteoid, and incorporation of normal fatty or hematopoietic marrow between the trabeculae (Figures 4-40 to 4-45).

Subungual exostosis is a subspecialized form of osteochondroma which appears on the terminal phalanx. It has a fibrocartilaginous component.

Intra-articular osteochondromas may also occur (dysplasia epiphysalis hemimelica). Osteochondromas of the articular surface are usually associated with multiple lesions, and cause severe early functional disturbance.

Malignant transformation of osteochondroma may occur when there is transformation of benign cartilaginous cap to chondrosarcoma, especially in axial skeleton. Any growth of the cartilaginous cap in a skeletally mature individual is suspicious.

OSTEOCHONDROMA

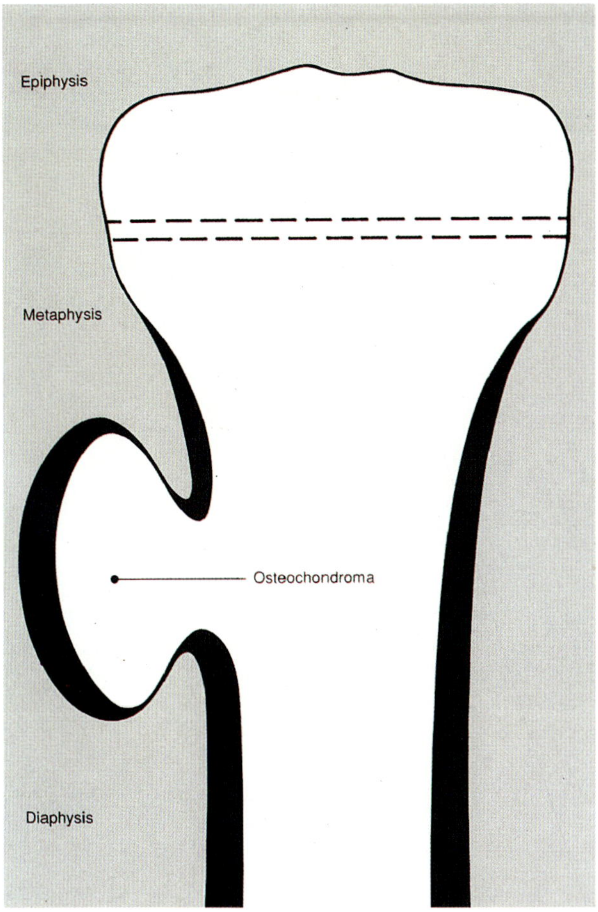

Figure 4-40. Radiographic manifestation, osteochondroma. The osteochondroma is an extension of the growth plate laterally. A cartilage cap is noted, transformation to bone is present underneath the cartilage cap, and the marrow cavity is incorporated into the proliferation of bone extending laterally. Osteochondromas may be pedunculated as illustrated, or sessile. The important histologic and radiographic manifestation is the incorporation of the marrow cavity into the stalk of the osteochondroma. This is in marked contrast to any of the juxtacortical tumors, including the benign periosteal chondroma. The cartilage cap of an osteochondroma should reflect the age of the individual. Any cartilage cap greater than 1 or 2 cm in an adult should be viewed with marked suspicion and probably indicates early transition to chondrosarcoma.

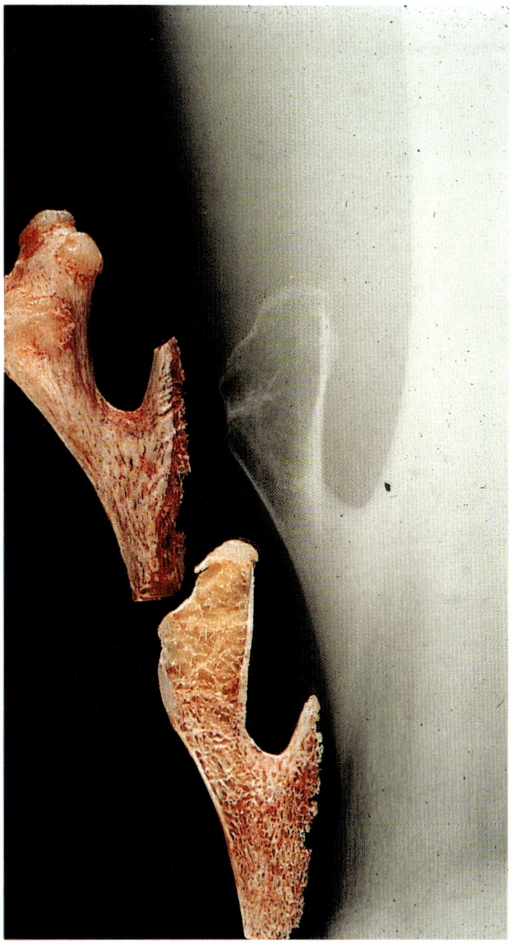

Figure 4-41. X-ray and specimen of an osteochondroma. Note the incorporation of the marrow into the stalk of the osteochondroma, and the extremely narrow cartilage cap remaining in this adult.

OSTEOCHONDROMA

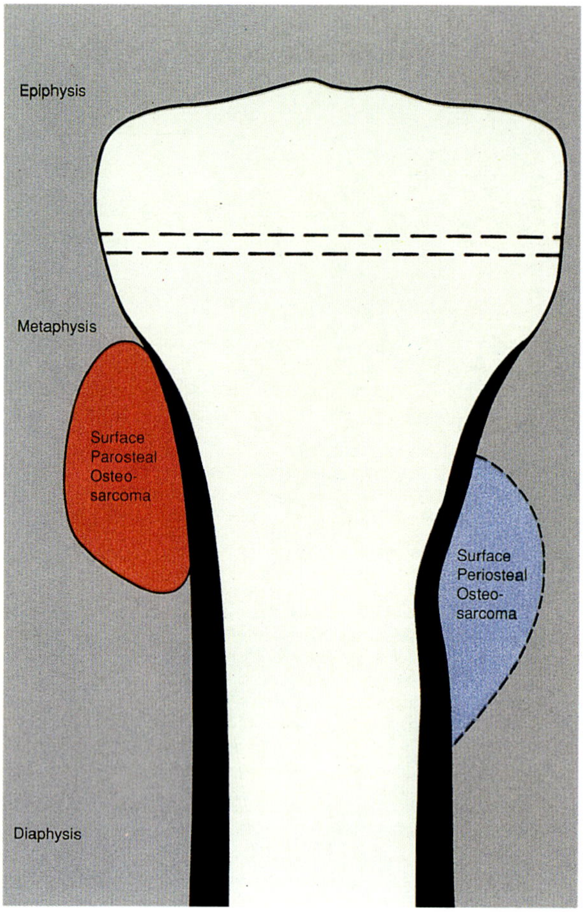

Figure 4-42. Schematic x-ray diagram of surface lesions. (See Figure 3-50).

Figure 4-43. Osteochondroma. The surface of an osteochondroma exhibiting the direct transition from perichondrium (periosteum) to cartilage. The origin of an osteochondroma is in the membrane surrounding the cap.

Figure 4-44. Osteochondroma. Primary trabecula formation in an osteochondroma. Note the acellular cartilage mimicking the primary trabecula that is normally seen at the growth plate, and the incorporation of normal marrow into the stalk of the osteochondroma.

Figure 4-45. Periosteal chondroma exhibiting moderate cellular variation and pleomorphism of the cartilage cells at the base of the lesion. A reactive rim of bone is present at the base, but there is no evidence of primary trabecula formation.

DIFFERENTIAL DIAGNOSIS OF OSTEOCHONDROMA

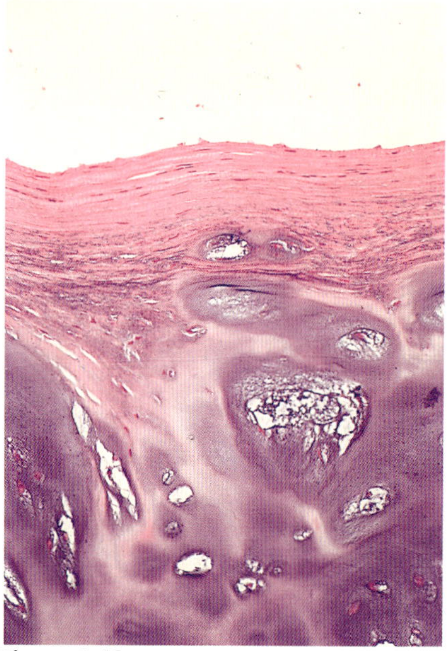

Figure 4-43.

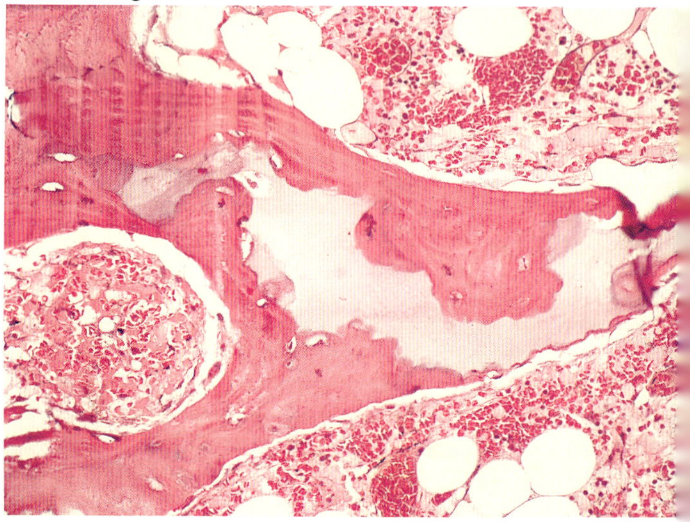

Figure 4-44.

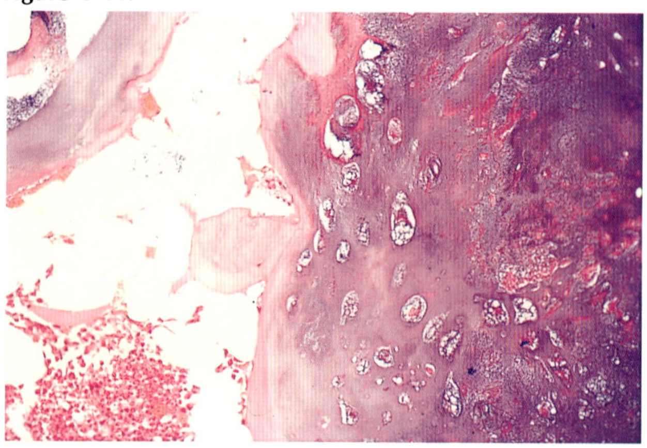

Figure 4-45.

REFERENCES

1. Dahlin DC, Salvador AH: Chondrosarcoma of bones of the hands and feet—study of 30 cases. *Cancer* 34:755–760, 1974.
2. Liu J, Hudkins PG, Swee RG, et al: Bone sarcomas associated with Ollier's disease. *Cancer* 59:1376–1385, 1987.
3. Nigrisoli M, Ferraro A, DeCristofaro R, et al: Chondrosarcoma of the hand and foot. *Chir Organi Mov* 75(4)315–323, 1990.
4. Welkerling H, Dreyer T, Delling G: Morphological typing of chondrosarcoma: A study of 94 cases. *Virchows Arch A Pathol Anat Histopathol* 418(5):419–425, 1991.
5. Gitelis S, Bertoni F, Picci P, et al: Chondrosarcoma of bone. J Bone Joint Surg 63A:1248–1257, 1981.
6. Healey JH, Lane LM: Chondrosarcoma. *Clin Orthop* 204: 119–130, 1986.
7. Ishida T, Kikuchi F, Machinami R: Histological grading and morphometric analysis of cartilaginous tumours. *Virchows Arch A Pathol Anat Histopathol* 418(2):149–155, 1991.
8. Bridge JA, Bhatia PS, Anderson JR, et al: Biologic and clinical significance of cytogenetic and molecular cytogenetic abnormalities in benign and malignant cartilaginous lesions. *Cancer Genet Cytogenet* 69(2):79–90, 1993.
9. Capanna R, Bertoni F, Bettelli G, et al: Dedifferentiated chondrosarcoma. *J Bone Joint Surg* 70A:69–79, 1988.
10. Daly PJ, Sim FH, Wold LE: Dedifferentiated chondrosarcoma of bone (clinical conference). *Orthopedics* 12(5): 763–767, 1989.
11. Frassica FJ, Unni KK, Beabout JW, et al: Dedifferentiated chondrosarcoma. *J Bone Joint Surg* 68A:1197–1205, 1986.
12. Bagley L, Kneeland JB, Dalinka MK, et al: Unusual behavior of clear cell chondrosarcoma. *Skeletal Radiol* 22(4): 279–282, 1993.
13. Present D, Bacchini P, Pignatti G, et al: Clear cell chondrosarcoma of bone. A report of 8 cases. *Skeletal Radiol* 20(3):187–191, 1991.
14. Bosse A, Ueda Y, Wuisman P, et al: Histogenesis of clear cell chondrosarcoma. An immunohistochemical study with osteonectin, a non-collagenous structure protein. *J Cancer Res Clin Oncol* 117(1):43–49, 1991.
15. Bertoni F, Picci P, Bacchini P, et al: Mesenchymal chondrosarcoma of bone and soft tissues. *Cancer* 52:533–541, 1983.
16. Swanson PE, Lillemoe TJ, Manivel JC, et al: Mesenchymal chondrosarcoma. An immunohistochemical study. *Arch Pathol Lab Med* 114(9):943–948, 1990.
17. Schajowicz F: *Tumors and Tumorlike Lesions of Bone. Pathology, Radiology, and Treatment.* Berlin, Springer-Verlag, 1994, pp 160–173, 189–201.
18. Walker WP, Landas SK, Bromley CM, et al: Immunohistochemical distinction of classic and chondroid chordomas. *Mod Pathol* 4(5):661–666, 1991.
19. Edel G, Ueda Y, Nakanishi J, et al: Chondroblastoma of bone. A clinical, radiological, light and immunohistochemical study. *Virchows Arch A Pathol Anat Histopathol* 421(4):355–366, 1992.
20. Turcotte RE, Kurt AM, Sim FH, et al: Chondroblastoma. *Hum Pathol* 24(9):944–949, 1993.

5

Differential Diagnosis of Intraosseous Lesions with Fibrous Connective Tissue

FIBROUS LESIONS

Fibrous Dysplasia

Fibrous dysplasia is an anomaly which arises at the growth plate of the developing child. Instead of the normal osteoblast, a spindled mesenchymal cell is produced which is incapable of forming the normal osseous structure. As a consequence the lesion is characterized by replacement of normal bone by a spindled cell proliferation accompanied by poorly formed (dysplastic) bone and occasional cartilage. Fibrous dysplasia replaces the normal trabecular bone, and may lead to deformity due to instability of the remaining bone. The disease exhibits various forms of expression. Monostotic fibrous dysplasia involves a single bone; the polyostotic form involves numerous bones, and Albright's syndrome is an endocrine disorder characterized by precocious puberty associated with skeletal lesions similar to fibrous dysplasia. Facial deformity may develop when skull bones are involved.

Because the lesion arises at the growth plate, the radiographic defect usually involves the full width of the tubular bone, lytic in the early lesion, but "ground glass" appearance as the lesion matures and becomes more heavily calcified (Figures 5-1, 5-2).[1]

The histologic picture consists of replacement of normal marrow and trabecular bone by spindled cellular elements. There is direct formation of poorly formed woven bone by the spindled fibrous tissue without an intervening osteoblastic layer. The bony trabeculae may be small, curved or slender "alphabet soup." Spherical deposits are usually present in the skull or flat bones. The stroma may contain rare foam-laden histiocytes and occasional giant cells. Foci of cartilage may be present.[2]

The lesion has been confused with osteofibrous dysplasia. Osteofibrous dysplasia is an intracortical lesion and exhibits a prominent rim of osteoblasts lining the trabeculae of bone. True fibrous dysplasia rarely has identifiable osteoblasts, but instead has direct transition from fibrous tissue to bone. The completely different and distinctive radiographic appearance of osteofibrous dysplasia should serve to separate the two entities.

The differential diagnosis of fibrous dysplasia must also include Paget's disease. In the lytic phase of Paget's disease there is replacement of the marrow by fibrous connective tissue, but there are always prominent osteoblasts and numerous osteoclasts, including the abnormally large "killer" osteoclasts.

Hyperparathyroidism may present a similar histologic picture, but it is a disseminated metabolic disease, so that all skeletal structures in the body are involved at the same time. A single lesion may exhibit fibrous replacement of focal portions of the bone, but other areas will exhibit normal hematopoietic and fatty marrow.

Although the differential diagnosis sounds fairly

DIFFERENTIAL DIAGNOSIS OF FIBROUS SKELETAL LESIONS

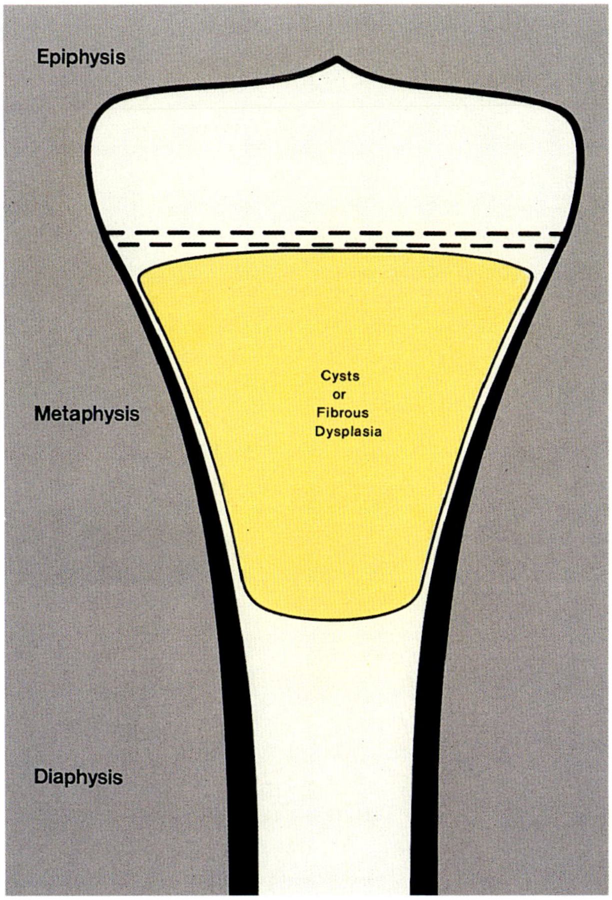

Figure 5-1. Fibrous dysplasia as well as the unicameral bone cyst arise at the growth plate, and usually extend completely across the bone early in its development. Thus, these lesions are characterized as central in location, rather than eccentric. Initially fibrous dysplasia is a purely lytic lesion with no evidence of bone formation and certainly no evidence of a periosteal reaction. As the lesion matures bone formation becomes apparent, and a "ground glass" pattern becomes prominent. "Ground glass" is not seen until the lesion matures and calcifies.

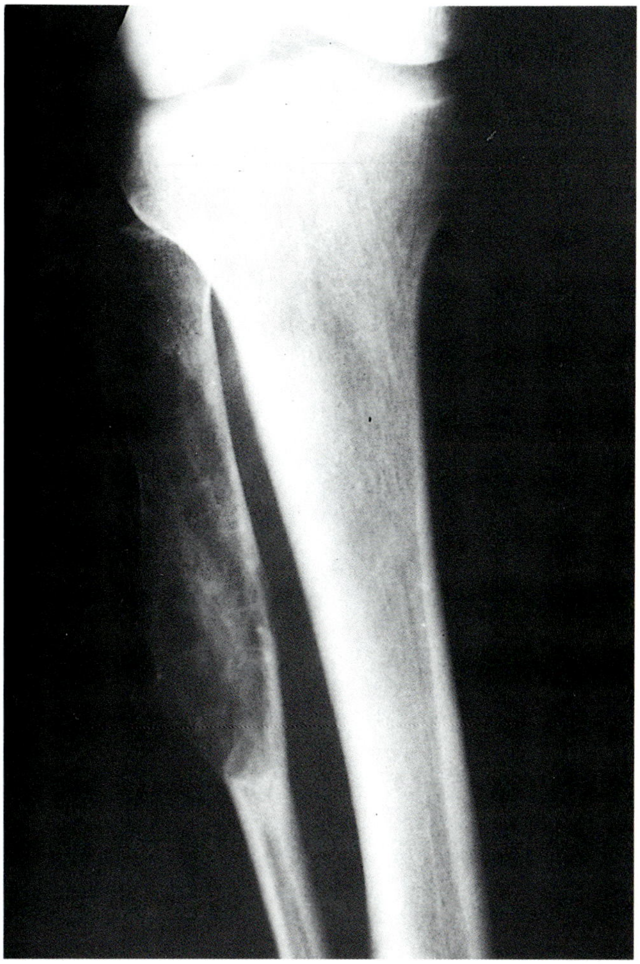

Figure 5-2. Centrally located lytic defect involving the full width of the bone. In this case the entire head of the fibula is involved in an elongated process.

straightforward, isolated fields of these entities can be confusing. One must keep the spectrum of differential diagnosis in mind when analyzing any single lesion with fibrous replacement of the marrow cavity (Figures 5-3 to 5-12).

The differential diagnosis must always include the well-differentiated intraosseous osteosarcoma. Often the pleomorphism or malignant characteristics of the well-differentiated osteosarcoma are not prominent, and the lesion is confused with a benign process, typically fibrous dysplasia. Careful attention to the uniform features of fibrous dysplasia, with extensive fibroblastic proliferation, primitive immature bone formation throughout the lesion, and usually, confinement of the fibrodysplastic process within the skeletal structure should help avoid the catastrophic mistake of confusing benign fibrous dysplasia with a well-differentiated intraosseous osteosarcoma.

In similar vein, the histologic appearance of a parosteal osteosarcoma may well present similar features to

DIFFERENTIAL DIAGNOSIS OF FIBROUS SKELETAL LESIONS

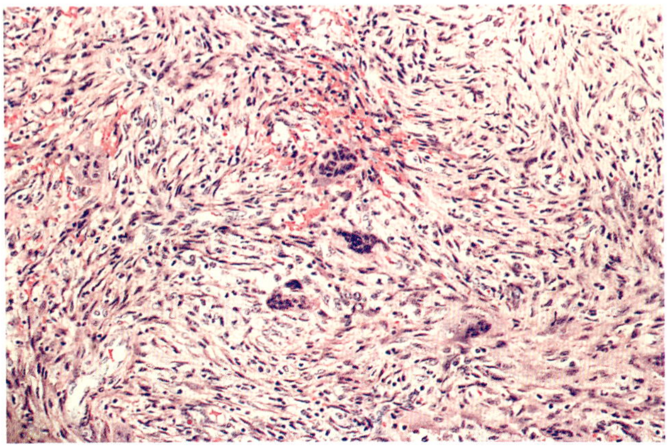

Figure 5-3. Nonossifying fibroma. Storiform pattern of fibroblasts, scattered giant cells, and an occasional xanthoma cell are present in this section. Note the absence of pleomorphism or mitotic activity.

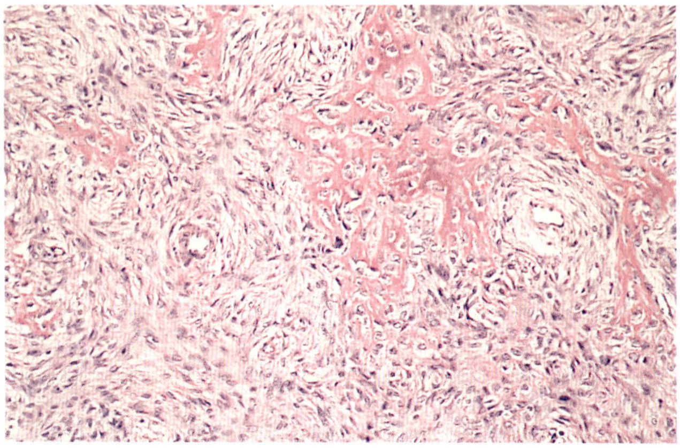

Figure 5-4. Fibrous dysplasia, early. The lesion exhibits marked cellularity of the fibrous component with early osteoid formation. Note the absence of osteoblasts lining the bone surface. There is direct transition from the fibroblast into the adjacent bony trabecula.

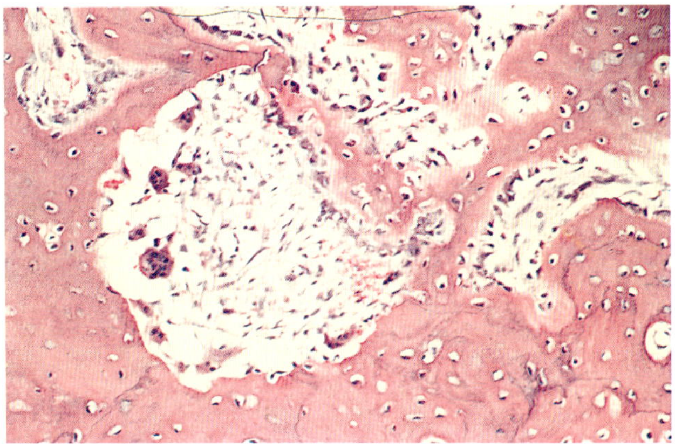

Figure 5-5. Hyperparathyroidism. Dissecting osteitis with replacement of the core of trabeculae of bone by unremarkable fibroblastic tissue. Note reinforcement of residual trabeculae by a seam of osteoblasts.

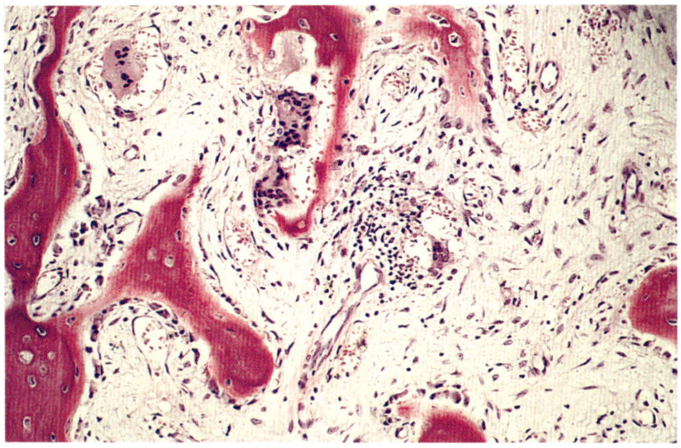

Figure 5-6. Paget's disease, lytic phase. Osteoclasts with unusually large number of nuclei, "killer osteoclasts," and numerous osteoblasts. The marrow has been replaced by nondescript fibrous connective tissue, and there are scattered foci of inflammatory cells.

DIFFERENTIAL DIAGNOSIS OF FIBROUS SKELETAL LESIONS

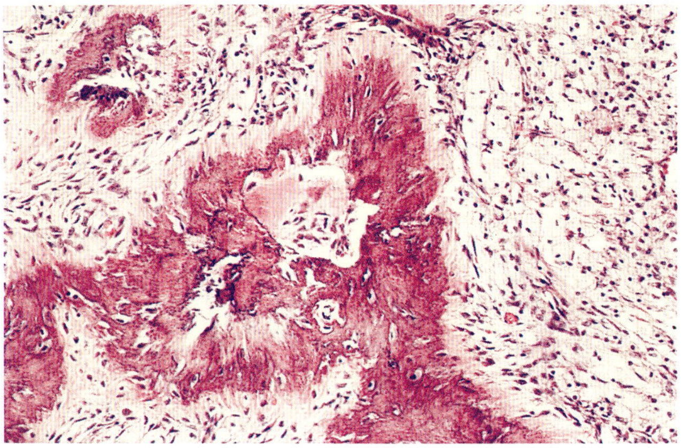

Figure 5-7. Nonossifying fibroma with calcification. Note the calcification pattern, the xanthoma cells, and fibroblasts.

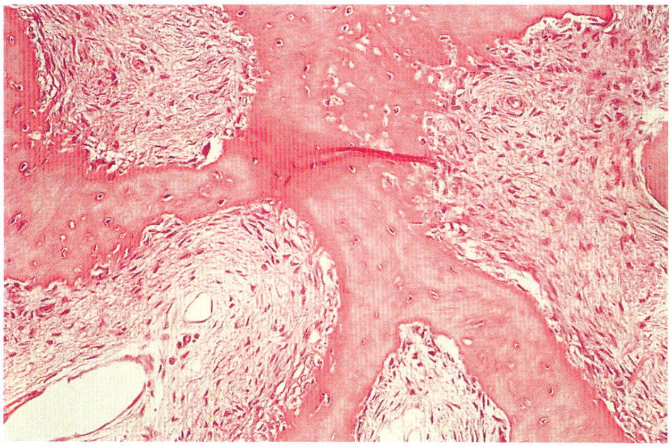

Figure 5-8. Fibrous dysplasia. More mature elements, with spindled fibroblasts and direct transition to trabecular bone. Although cells are present at the interface between the fibrous connective tissue and the bone, these are not the normal plump osteoblasts lining a normal trabecular surface.

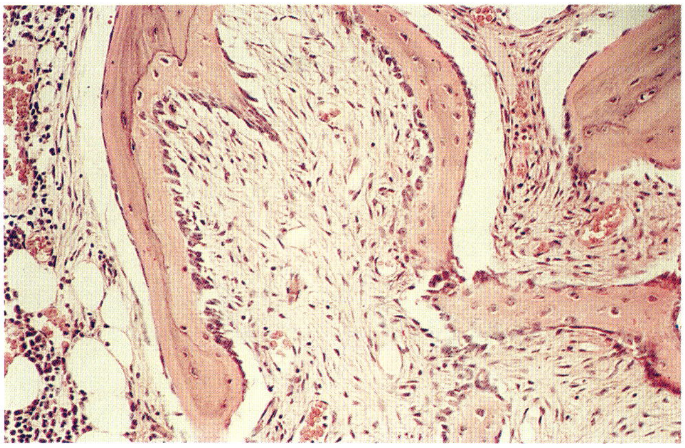

Figure 5-9. Hyperparathyroidism. Dissecting osteitis with replacement of the core of trabecula of bone by unremarkable fibroblastic tissue. Note reinforcement of residual trabeculae by a seam of osteoblasts. (Normal marrow is present adjacent to the dissecting osteitis.)

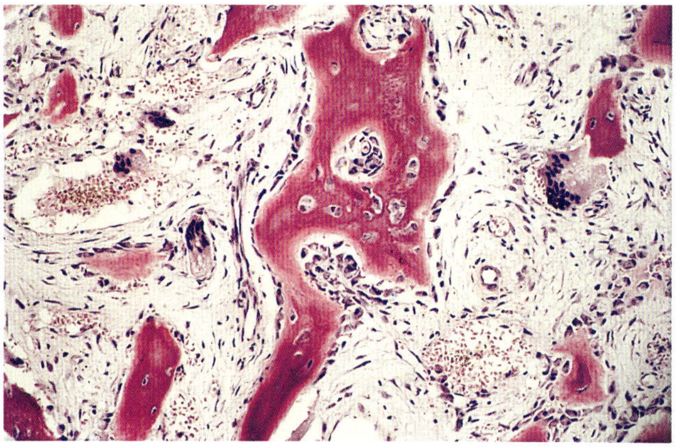

Figure 5-10. Paget's disease, lytic phase. Killer osteoclasts, extensive osteoblast activity, fibrous replacement of normal marrow, and numerous dilated vascular channels.

DIFFERENTIAL DIAGNOSIS OF FIBROUS SKELETAL LESIONS

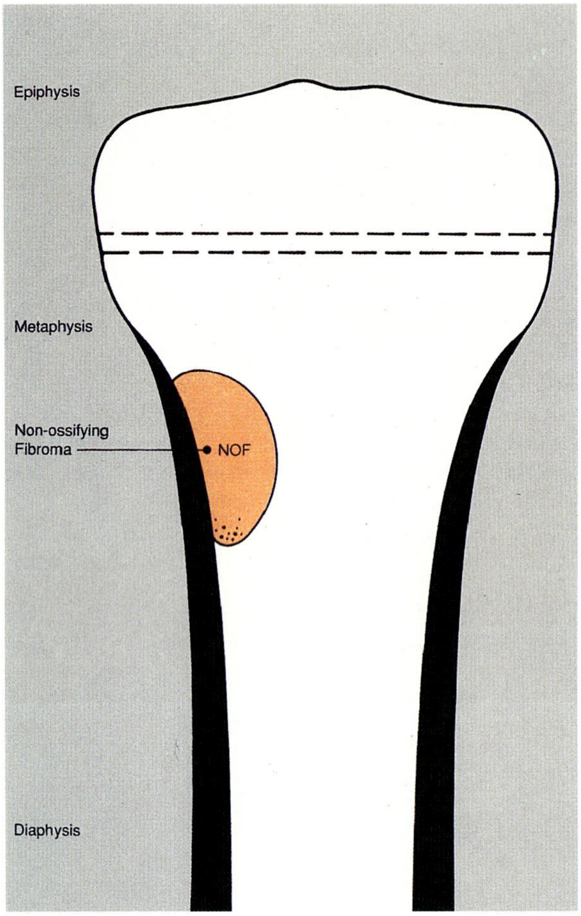

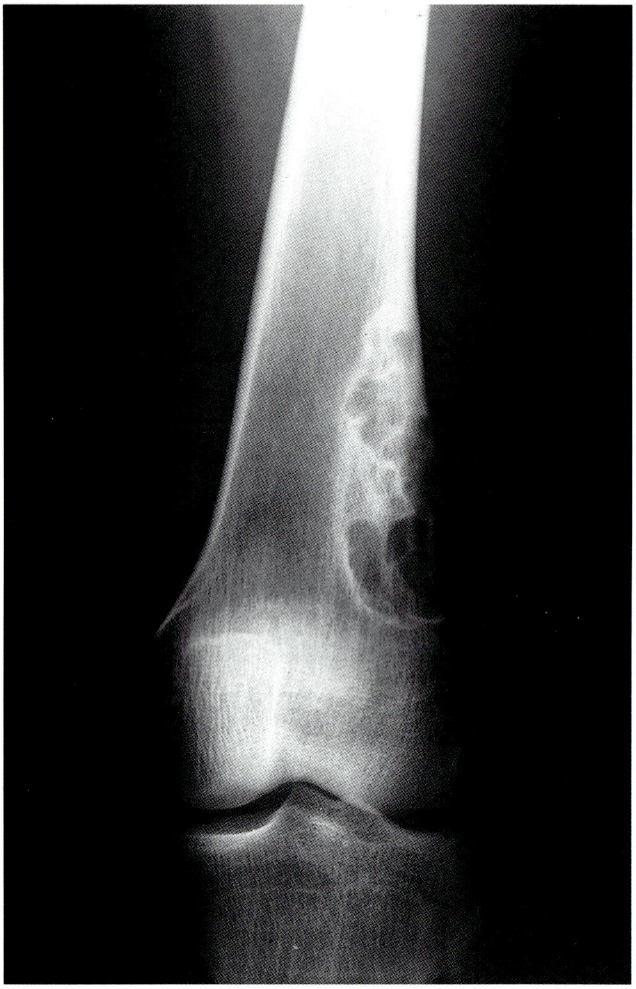

Figures 5-11, 5-12. Nonossifying fibroma. Eccentric sharply circumscribed lytic defect, metaphyseal, usually at some distance from the growth plate. The older portion of the lesion (the most metaphyseal or diaphyseal) may exhibit foci of calcification, as in this case. No periosteal reaction is visible.

fibrous dysplasia. This mistake can only be made when one ignores the radiographic presentation.

Nonossifying Fibroma

Nonossifying fibroma may start as a metaphyseal intracortical defect composed of fibrous connective tissue and expand slowly. The cortex of the normal child grows laterally at a faster rate than the tumor, thus during normal development the lesion slowly migrates into the medullary portion of the metaphysis. Older lesions calcify, subsequently ossify and are remodeled into the normal trabecular pattern. Remodeling is the basis of the disappearance, but lesions must calcify and then ossify to be remodeled.

The radiographic appearance is almost completely diagnostic. The lesion is a metaphyseal defect, circumscribed, eccentrically located, with or without a rim of reactive bone (Figures 5-11, 5-12).

The histology consists of whorled storiform fibrous tissue with a cartwheel pattern, numerous xanthoma cells (foam-laden histiocytes), numerous giant cells, and little if any pleomorphism or mitotic activity.

Under normal circumstances, the nonossifying fibroma slowly calcifies, then forms bone in the area of calcification, and the bone is remodeled into the trabecular pattern of the host bone. The lesion belongs in the category of "don't touch lesions," with certain exceptions.[3]

The early nonossifying fibroma should be differentiated from the subperiosteal metaphyseal defect, or cortical desmoid (Armed Forces Institute of Pathology). This defect arises at the linea aspera at the insertion of the adductor magnus as subperiosteal defect secondary to unusual stress or muscular activity in a skeletally immature individual. The lesions are often bilateral and heal spontaneously. (See p 11.)

Osteofibrous Dysplasia

The osteofibrous dysplasia of long bone is a rare lesion, usually located in either the tibia or fibula, where it may present as single or multiple intracortical lesions. Despite statistical prevalence in these two bones, there are occasional case reports with locations in other structures, including ulna, radius, and vertebral bodies.[4,5]

Radiographically, the lesion is lytic, located entirely within the cortex, with sharply demarcated intracortical margins slowly expanding the external and internal margin of the cortex. The classical lesion should not extend into the medullary cavity; when it does, one should suspect the presence of an adamantinoma. The histologic pattern resembles fibrous dysplasia. However, the trabeculae are lined by a distinct rim of osteoblasts. The intracortical location and osteoblastic seam differentiate it from classical fibrous dysplasia (Figures 5-13 to 5-15). Superficial similarity to early lytic Paget's disease may be a source of confusion. Although an occasional osteoclast can be seen in the connective tissue stroma, the osteoclasts are small and normal as opposed to the large "killer" osteoclasts of Paget's disease (Figures 5-6, 5-10).

Adamantinoma of Long Bone

The tumor is similar in location to osteofibrous dysplasia but demonstrates a more aggressive growth pattern.

The location of the tumor is usually diaphyseal, with an intracortical component, expansion to involve medullary cavity, and varying evidence of aggressive behavior. On the whole, lesions tend to be low grade.

The histology consists of two components including a fibrous component similar to osteofibrous dysplasia, but an additional component consisting of epithelioid clusters which react with immunohistochemical stains for epithelial elements. Transition from osteofibrous dysplasia to adamantinoma has been documented in the literature (Figures 5-16 to 5-19).[5–10]

The adamantinoma is a malignant tumor, with relatively low biologic potential. In those rare cases where metastases are present, it is the epithelioid component which metastasizes, without the accompanying fibrous elements (Figures 5-13 to 5-15).

Desmoplastic Fibroma and Desmoplastic Fibrosarcoma

The desmoplastic fibroma is a rare intraosseous neoplasm with which there is a profusion of fibroblasts forming dense heavily collagenized connective tissue. The lesion should show a sharply circumscribed margin, and no evidence of aggressive growth on radiographic analysis. The histology is characterized by spindled fibroblasts and dense collagenization. Mitotic figures and nuclear pleomorphism should be absent.[11,12]

Desmoplastic fibromas tend to calcify, and thus mimic an osteoblastic lesion in radiographic appearance. It is important to differentiate calcification of soft tissue from bona fide osteoid formation by a neoplasm. By definition, a fibroma does not form osteoid.

The desmoplastic fibrosarcoma is the same fibrous tumor exhibiting pleomorphism and mitotic activity, with malignant radiographic and histologic characteristics. Again the lesion may calcify, but bone formation by the tumor cell should be absent. An aggressive growth pattern is prevalent, and occasionally the lesion dedifferentiates into a full-blown fibrosarcoma. Fortunately, both the desmoplastic fibroma and the desmoplastic fibrosarcoma are relatively rare lesions. It is often difficult to differentiate between the benign and malignant desmoplastic lesion, and wide excision for both is therefore an appropriate recommendation (Figures 5-20 to 5-22).

Malignant Fibrous Histiocytoma

Malignant fibrous histiocytoma is a primary tumor of bone with a pleomorphic neoplastic proliferation including fibrous and histiocytic elements.

The radiographic presentation consists of a poorly defined lytic destructive process with a moth-eaten or permeative pattern of destruction; periosteal reaction may be present. The radiographic appearance does not help to differentiate the lesion from other noncalcified matrix-producing malignant tumors of bone.

As opposed to the pure fibrosarcoma of bone, a malignant fibrous histiocytoma is characterized by a storiform whorled pattern with greater pleomorphism of the tumor cell. Fibroblasts and lipid-laden tumor cells are present in the lesion. Multinucleated and giant tumor cells are

DIFFERENTIAL DIAGNOSIS OF FIBROUS SKELETAL LESIONS

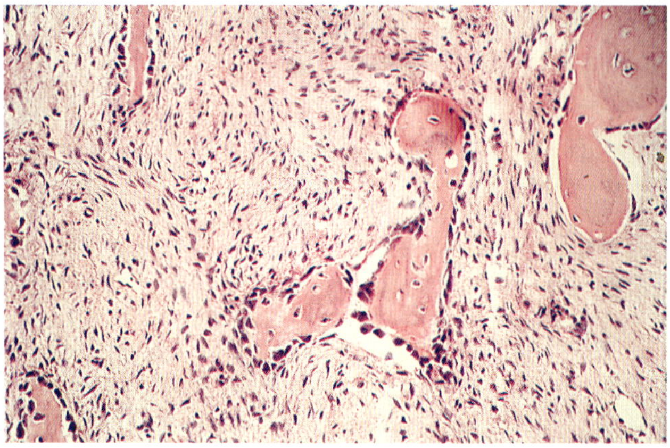

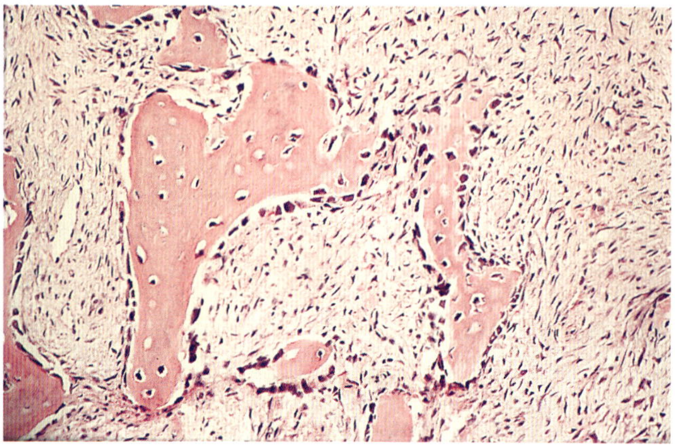

Figures 5-13, 5-14. Osteofibrous dysplasia. Note the prominent osteoblastic seam lining the immature trabeculae of bone, accompanied by fibroblastic tissue. These osteoblasts serve to differentiate the osteofibrous dysplasia from the true centrally located fibrous dysplasia of bone.

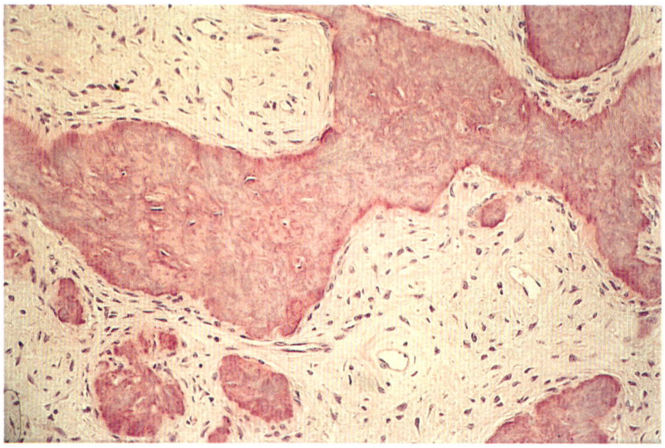

Figure 5-15. Fibrous dysplasia. Less cellular fibrous connective tissue, indicating maturity of the process with the formation of immature bone fragments. The bone always retains its woven pattern under polarized light.

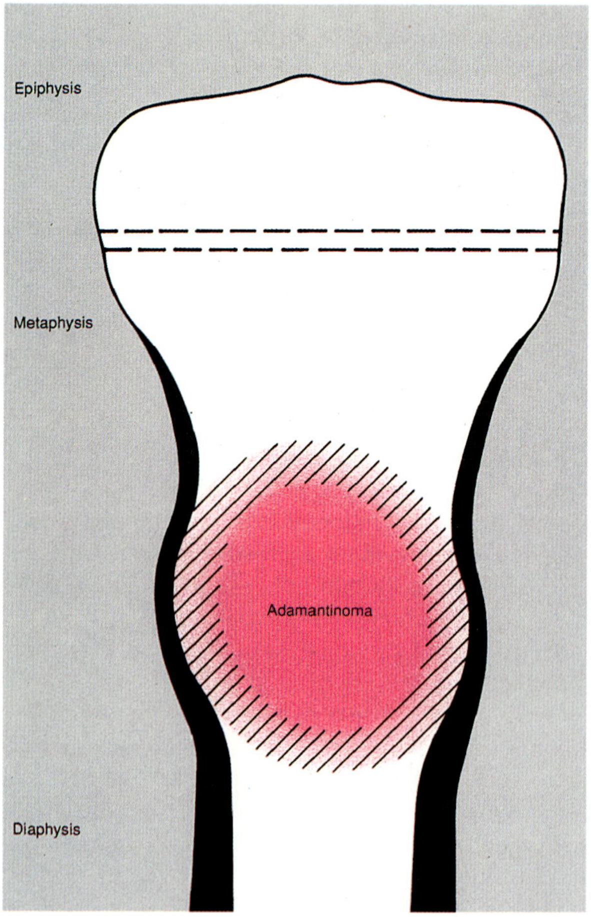

Figure 5-16. The adamantinoma of long bone is an intracortical and intramedullary tumor, causing scalloping of the internal margin with some indistinct moth-eaten margin of the lesion within the bone. As a rule these lesions do not produce a permeative pattern or a periosteal reaction, but they are capable of metastasis, and therefore have to be considered a low grade malignant neoplasm.

DIFFERENTIAL DIAGNOSIS OF FIBROUS SKELETAL LESIONS

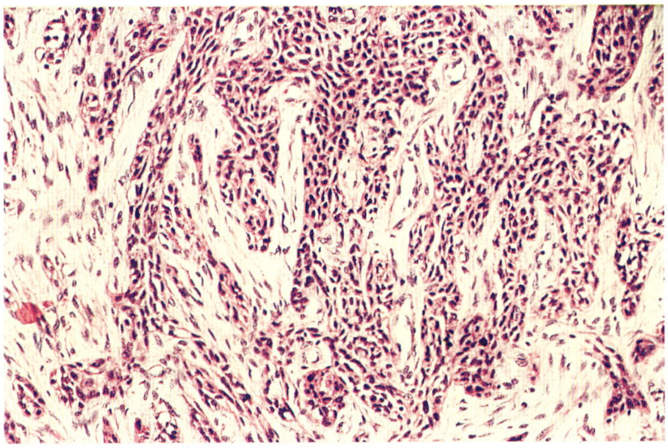

Figure 5-17. Adamantinoma of long bone. Clusters of epithelioid cells surrounded by a fibrous connective tissue component. This pattern is characteristic of the biphasic nature of an adamantinoma. The possibility of metastatic carcinoma must always be considered when viewing this lesion.

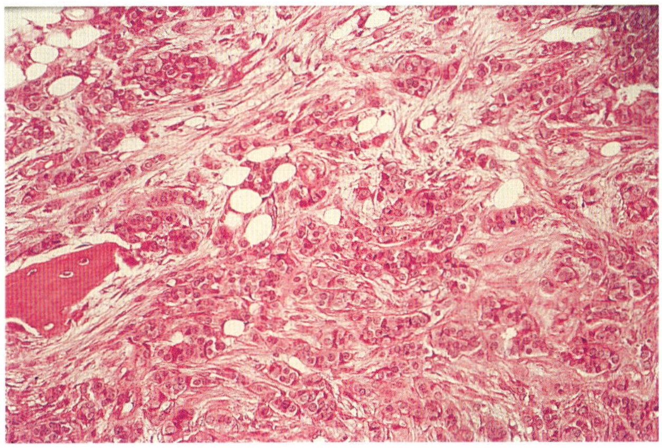

Figure 5-18. Metastatic carcinoma (primary carcinoma of prostate).

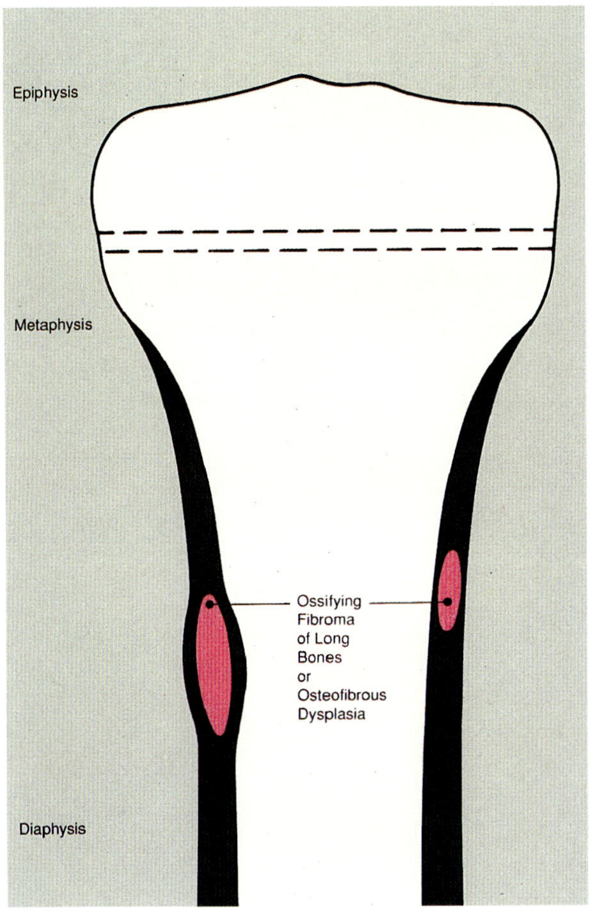

Figure 5-19. Osteofibrous dysplasia. These lesions are intracortical, usually diaphyseal, and expand both sides of the cortex. Because x-rays are two-dimensional studies, the appearance of these lesions may be misleading, and one may be misled into assuming that the lesion is within the medullary cavity. Careful radiographic positioning, however, will demonstrate the intracortical nature of these processes.

common. There is no evidence of osteoid formation by the tumor cell.[13]

These tumors have been associated with previous benign bone lesions, including infarcts, cysts, Paget's disease, and previously irradiated bone. This entity has been described as a separate classifiable tumor of bone since 1972 (Figures 5-23 to 5-28).

Fibrosarcoma

The primary fibrosarcoma of bone is a malignant intraosseous tumor of fibroblasts.

The radiographic appearance is one of a poorly defined lesion usually found in the metaphysis, with either moth-eaten or permeative destruction. There is a tendency to infarct trabecular fragments of bone. The presence or absence of a periosteal reaction depends upon rate of tumor growth.

The histology consists of moderately pleomorphic fibroblasts with extensive mitotic activity. The tumor will form fairly uniform interwoven bands of collagen with a characteristic "herringbone" pattern. The ground sub-

DIFFERENTIAL DIAGNOSIS OF FIBROUS SKELETAL LESIONS

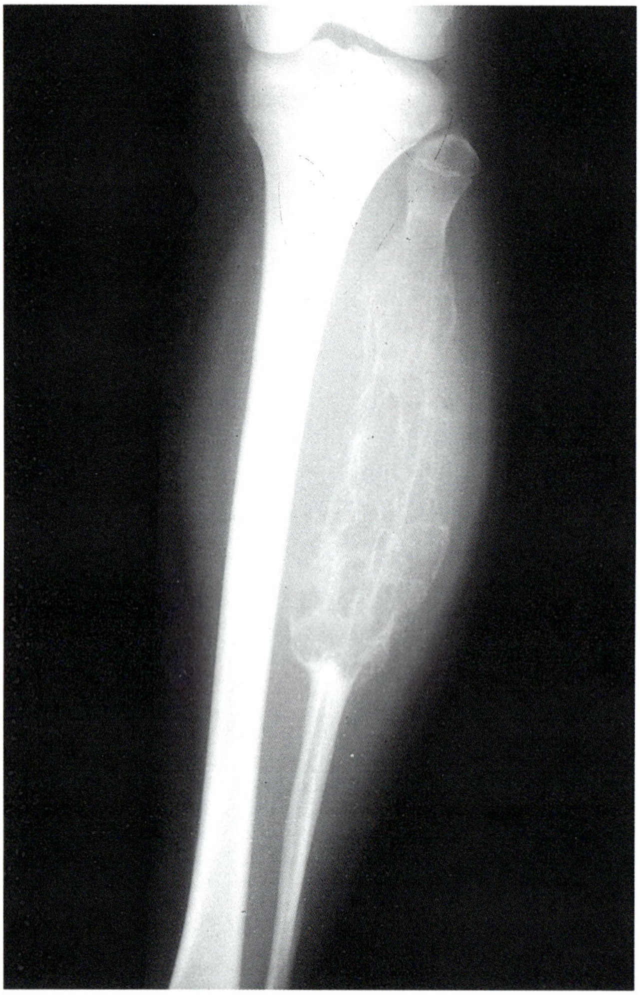

Figure 5-20. Desmoplastic fibroma. The lesion is sharply circumscribed, completely destroying the proximal portion of the fibula and expanding into the adjacent soft tissue. However, there is a sharp margin in both the proximal and distal portion of the lesion, indicating its slow growth potential.

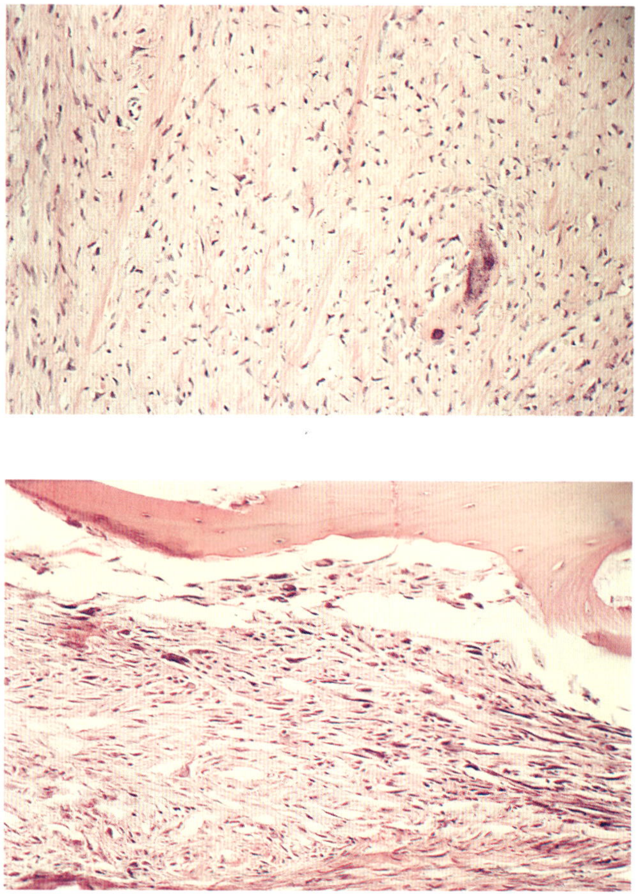

Figures 5-21, 5-22. Desmoplastic fibroma (Figure 5-21) and fibrosarcoma (Figure 5-22). Note the extensive collagen formation by the lesion, the focal areas of calcification within the fibrous component, and uniform spindled fibroblasts, exhibiting pleomorphism in the case of the sarcoma. Desmoplastic fibromas and desmoplastic fibrosarcomas have a tendency to calcify.

DIFFERENTIAL DIAGNOSIS OF FIBROUS SKELETAL LESIONS

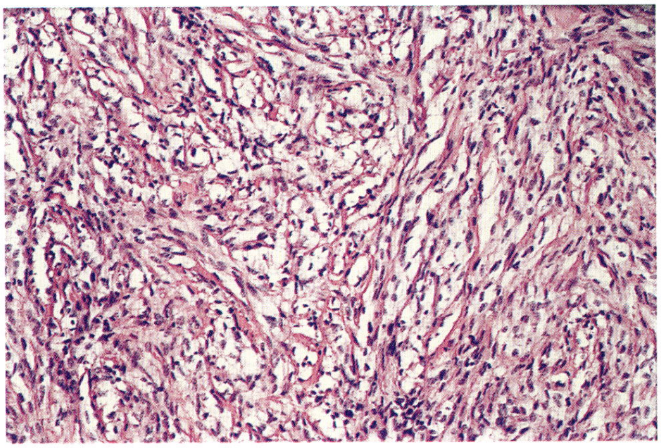

Figure 5-23. Metastatic renal cell carcinoma. Note the clear cell pattern prevalent in the midst of what appear to be spindled cells but in reality are spindled epidermal cancer cells. Again the clear cells may be confused with a histiocytic tumor, and misinterpreted as xanthoma cells. Immunohistochemistry will readily resolve the issue.

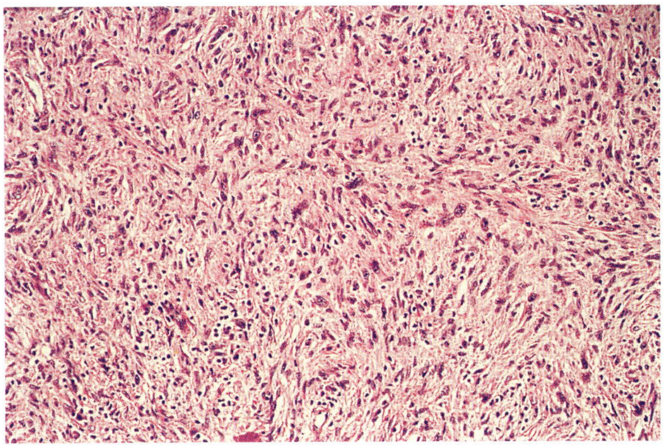

Figure 5-24. Malignant fibrous histiocytoma. The storiform pattern is readily apparent. There is moderate pleomorphism, and variation in nuclear size and staining.

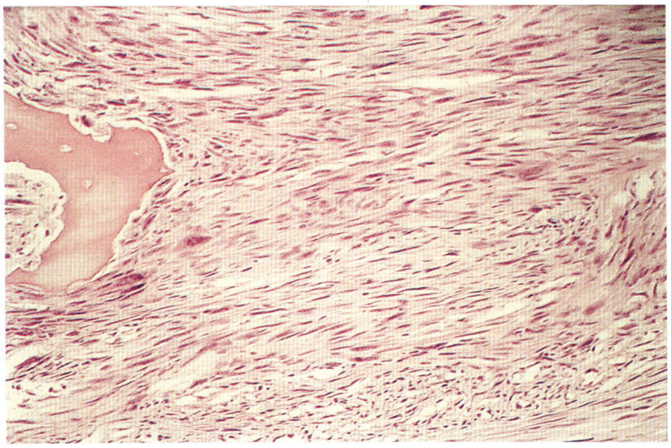

Figure 5-25. Fibrosarcoma of bone. There is a herringbone pattern with moderate nuclear pleomorphism and hyperchromatic nuclei. The permeative pattern is apparent by its relationship to the adjacent bone.

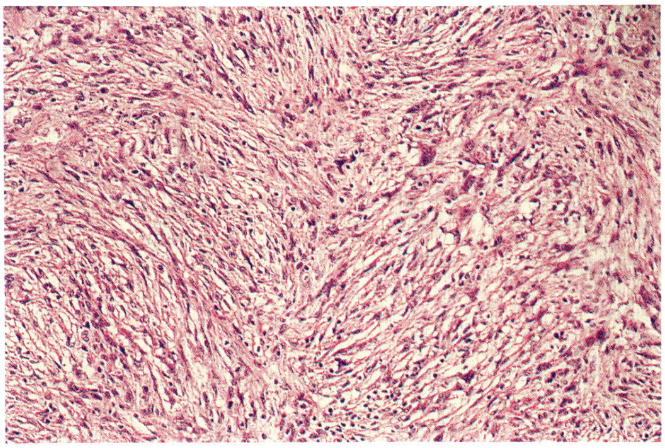

Figure 5-26. Nonossifying fibroma. .Storiform pattern of fibrous proliferation, with minimal variation in nuclear size and staining, scattered giant cells, and numerous xanthoma cells.

DIFFERENTIAL DIAGNOSIS OF FIBROUS SKELETAL LESIONS

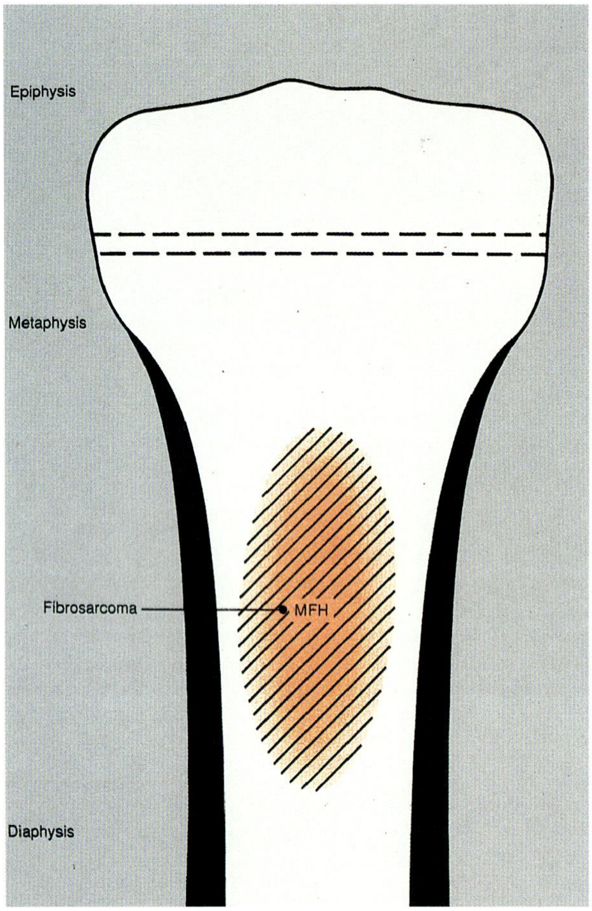

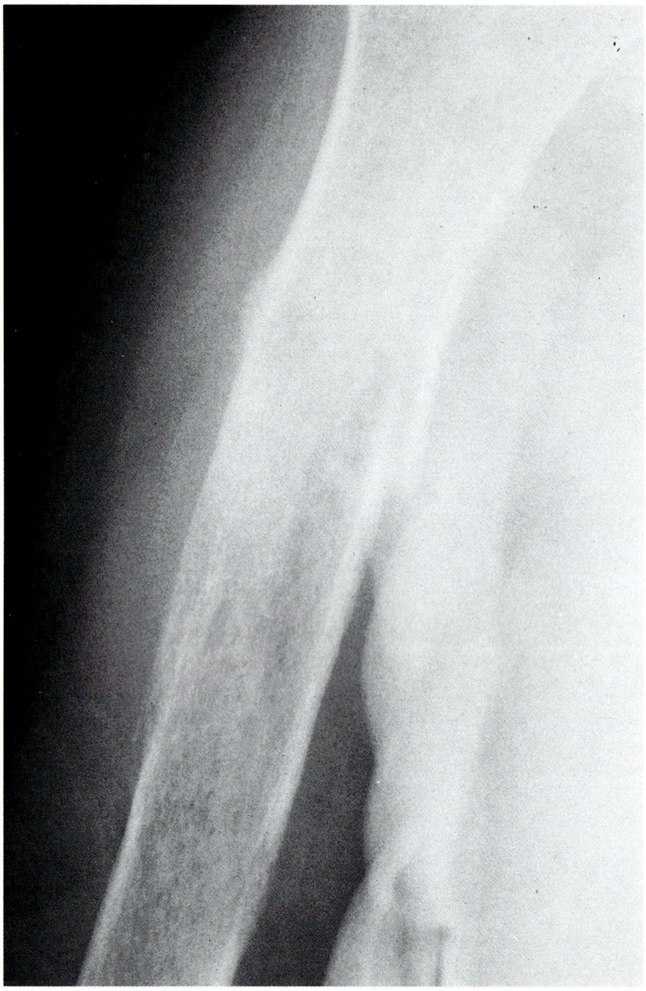

Figures 5-27, 5-28. Malignant fibrous histiocytoma or fibrosarcoma. These lesions are lytic, poorly defined, either permeative or moth-eaten destructive patterns, with or without periosteal reactions. However, they should never produce identifiable matrix calcification. As a rule the MFH as well as the fibrosarcoma is found in the metaphyseal or diaphyseal portion of the long bone.

stance consists of collagen, but the tumor does not form identifiable osteoid (Figure 5-22).

Many cases exhibit difficulty in differentiating a primary fibrosarcoma of bone from a malignant fibrous histiocytoma. There is really no practical point to the differentiation. Both lesions are primarily composed of fibrous connective tissue, exhibit histologic features of malignancy, and should not have either cartilage or osseous matrix formation by the tumor. In the classical case the fibrosarcoma is usually better differentiated with identifiable spindle cells, herringbone pattern with alternating direction of fiber growth, and a lack of markedly pleomorphic cells, as opposed to malignant fibrous histiocytoma. Classical manifestations of fibrosarcoma are encroachment into the trabecular bone and infarction of small trabeculae. At this time preoperative and postoperative management, chemotherapy and surgical approaches to malignant fibrous histiocytoma and fibrosarcoma are the same.

CYSTIC LESIONS

Unicameral Bone Cyst

The unicameral bone cyst arises at the growth plate of the developing child. The abnormality results in the loss

DIFFERENTIAL DIAGNOSIS OF CYSTIC LESIONS OF THE SKELETON

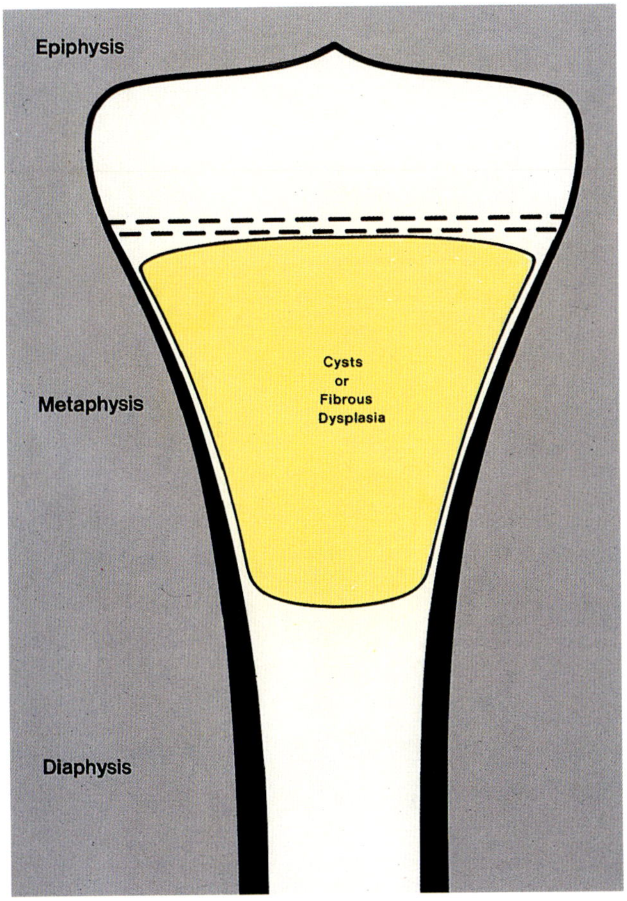

Figure 5-29. The unicameral bone cyst arises at an early age at the growth plate, and as the child grows the growth plate may or may not grow away from the lesion. Thus with an open growth plate the lesion is always metaphyseal. It is usually centrally located, with a lytic component and sharply defined margins. In cases of fracture there may be a periosteal reaction; but on the whole, without trauma, the unicameral bone cyst does not elicit any periosteal reaction. Fragments of bone may be caught within the cyst, and because of the fluid nature of the cyst cavity these fragments may float and change their position depending upon the position of the bone. This "falling leaf" sign identifies the fluid nature of the cyst content.

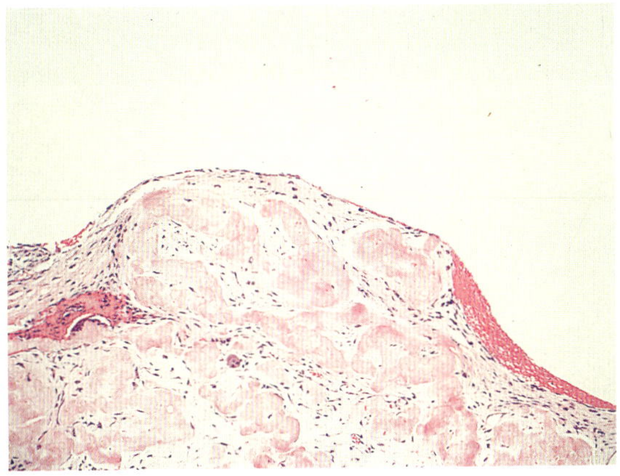

Figure 5-30. Unicameral bone cyst. Note the mesothelial lining, the formation of "cementum-like" bone just beneath the cyst lining. The cementum-like bone consists of masses of osteoid without osteocytic lacunae.

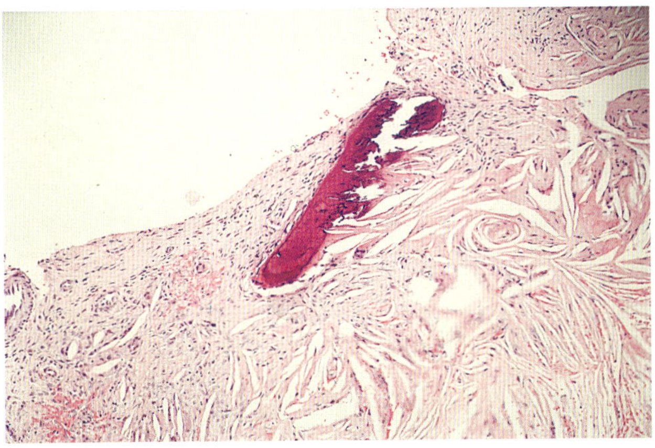

Figure 5-31. Unicameral bone cyst. Numerous cholesterol clefts, a fragment of reactive bone in the wall of the cyst, and fibrous connective tissue.

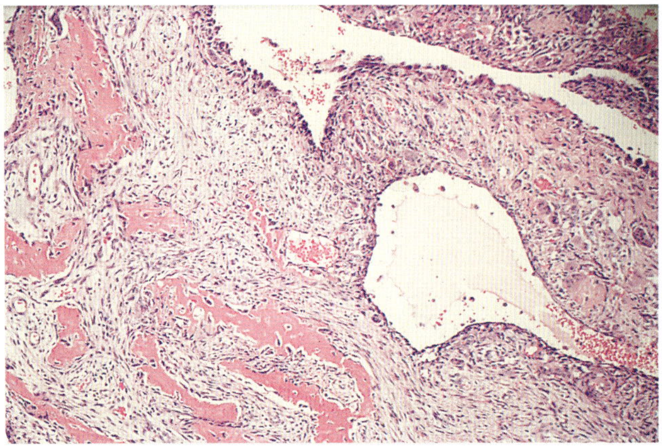

Figure 5-32. Aneurysmal bone cyst. A cavity with blood, a semblance of an endothelial lining. If examined at higher magnification one can establish that these are simply fibroblasts or giant cells lining up along the edge of the cavity. Reinforcement of the cavity by immature reactive bone.

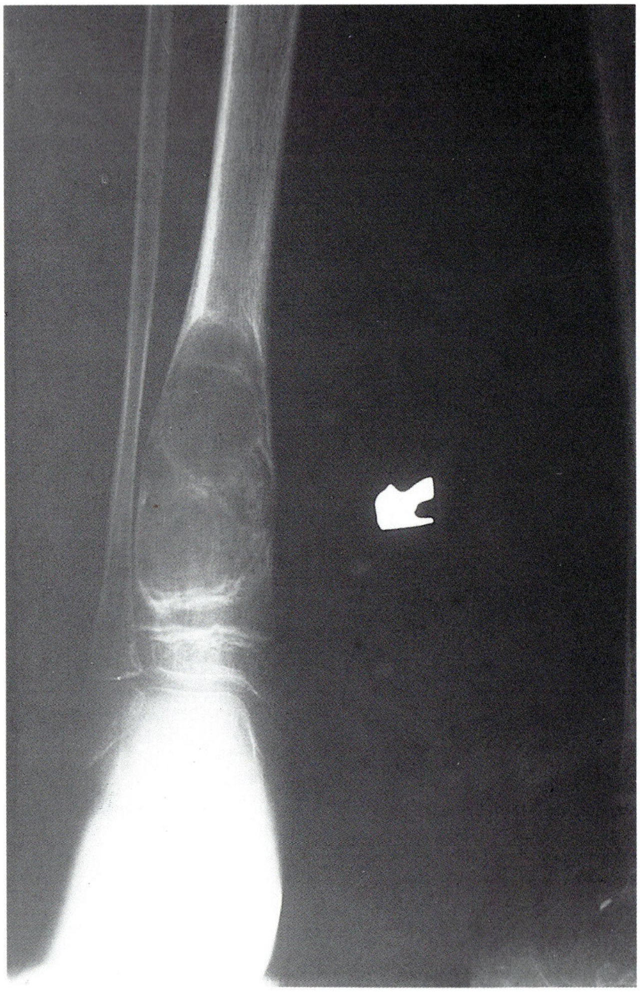

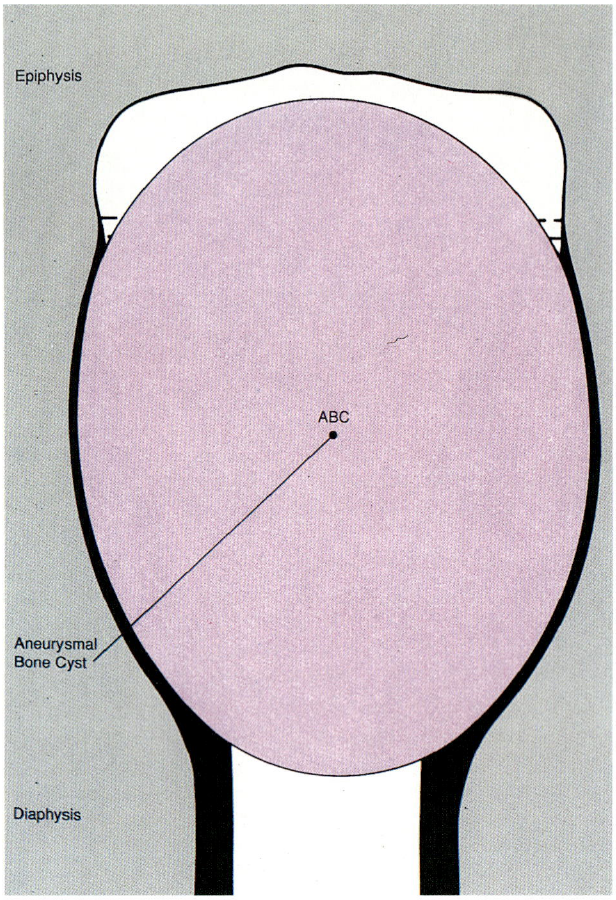

Figures 5-33, 5-34. The aneurysmal bone cyst is filled with blood. It may aggressively expand the bone, but usually has a very sharp margin, and unless fracture results, does not usually have periosteal reaction. These expansile lesions may be quite extensive, and balloon the bone beyond its original contour. As a rule the aneurysmal bone cyst is filled with blood and does not contain identifiable calcifiable matrix.

DIFFERENTIAL DIAGNOSIS OF CYSTIC LESIONS OF THE SKELETON

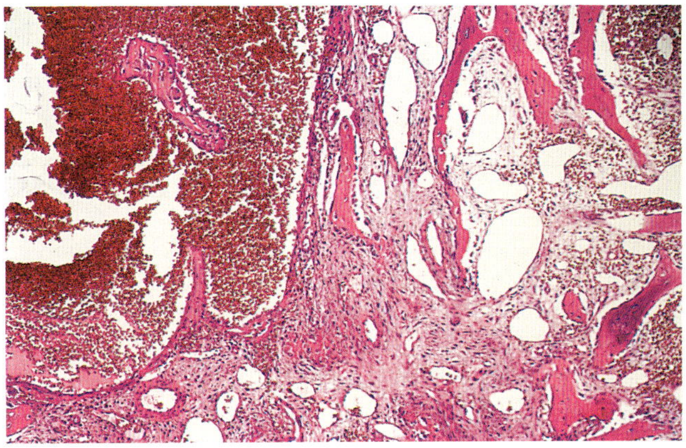

Figure 5-35. Aneurysmal bone cyst. Blood-filled cavity, no vessel lining, reinforcement by thin trabeculae of reactive bone.

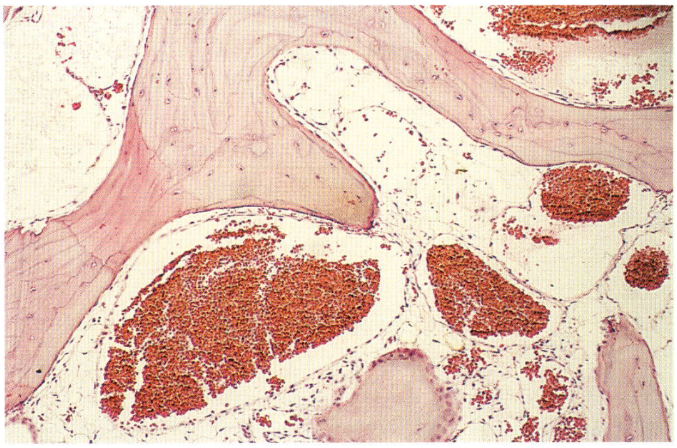

Figure 5-36. Angioma of bone. As opposed to the aneurysmal bone cyst, there is an identifiable vessel lining, and trabecular reinforcement of bone fragments.

of the bone-forming cells, with undifferentiated mesenchymal components replacing normal bone formation. This undifferentiated or "uncommitted metaphyseal lesion"[14] goes on to develop myxoid characteristics, ultimately resulting in the formation of a cyst. Because the lesion is an anomaly arising at the growth plate, the lesion is usually a sharply circumscribed metaphyseal lesion quick to involve the full diameter of the involved bone. The margins are sharply defined. Unless fractured, there is no periosteal reaction. An active lesion is in contact with the epiphyseal growth plate. At certain times, for no apparent discernible reason, the lesion ceases to be active, and the growth plate may grow away from the lesion, relocating the cyst further toward the diaphyseal portion of the long bone.

The histology of the unicameral bone cyst consists of a single layered mesothelium with underlying connective tissue and some reactive bone formation at the margin of the cyst. Cholesterol clefts, hemosiderin deposits, and focal areas of dense fibrous connective tissue are often associated with the cyst. Neoplastic bone formation (cementum-like bone) is a feature of older cysts and consists of masses of osteoid with a lining of spindle-shaped osteoblasts. Osteocytes encased in lacunar spaces are rare, hence the similarity to cementum. On rare occasions the fibrous connective tissue and neoplastic bone formation may lead to malignant transformation (malignant fibrous histiocytoma) (Figures 5-29 to 5-31).

The unicameral bone cyst has been successfully treated with steroid injection, described by Campanacci et al.[15] Success varies, but inactive cysts respond better than active cysts; in the most recent publication, a 74% success rate is claimed for those lesions located in the diaphysis. Additional favorable factors for steroid therapy include unilocular versus multilocular cysts, and smaller versus larger size of the lesion itself.

The differential diagnosis includes subarticular cyst formation in osteoarthritis. Under those circumstances cysts may be formed in close proximity to a major joint. They represent increased turnover of articular cartilage with deposition of myxoid material in the subchondral area leading to chondrogranuloma, liquefaction, and ultimately cyst formation. This should not be confused with unicameral bone cysts.

Early antibiotic therapy may result in aborted osteomyelitis which in turn may leave a fluid-filled cavity with only an occasional inflammatory cell. One should consider the diagnosis when a cyst presents in an atypical location (epiphysis).

Aneurysmal Bone Cyst

The aneurysmal bone cyst is a vascular lesion consisting of widely dilated vascular channels which are not lined by any identifiable endothelium. They may grow rapidly and may destroy bone by rapid expansion and pressure.[16]

The radiographic appearance consists of a lesion which is expansile, lytic, and sharply circumscribed. Although a rapidly growing lesion may create a periosteal reaction with a Codman triangle, the margins should stabilize at some point. The division of aneurysmal bone cyst into aggressive, active, and inactive lesions is based upon the radiographic appearance. An aggressive lesion is one that expands and exhibits an incomplete, poorly defined rim or periosteal reaction. An active lesion is one in which the reactive new bone only forms a partial shell. An inactive lesion exhibits a complete rim of reactive new bone.

The lesions may be found in various locations; they have been defined by Campanacci et al.[15] as four different types, depending upon their location. Type I lesions are located in the center of a long bone, type II lesions actually expand the diameter of the bone, and are usually found in the smaller, thinner bones such as fibula and radius; type III lesions are eccentric intraosseous lesions, and type IV are subperiosteal.[17] Occasional solid lesions may be found.

Unlike the unicameral bone cyst, the aneurysmal bone cyst does not respond to intracavitary injection of cortisone. Surgery is the acceptable method of therapy, and aggressive cysts should be widely curetted with postoperative phenol or cryosurgery. Radiation therapy should be avoided unless the lesion is inaccessible. Unfortunately, numerous aneurysmal bone cysts are located in the vertebral column and cannot be easily treated with surgery.

The histology is variable. The aneurysmal bone cyst is a cystic cavity, and the cyst should be filled with blood. The wall of the cyst may contain a variable number of giant cells, fibrous connective tissue, and osteoblasts forming reactive bones. Giant cells are located near the edge of the cyst (Figures 5-32 to 5-35).

The lesion has been associated with a benign unicameral bone cyst, giant cell tumor of bone, chondroblastoma, chondromyxoid fibroma, osteoblastoma, osteosarcoma, and numerous other lesions.

The differential diagnosis must include a lytic telangiectatic osteosarcoma. The wall of the sarcoma contains clearly identifiable sarcomatous elements. Hemangiomas of bone consist of true vessels with an endothelial lining (Figure 5-36).

In the opinion of many observers, the aneurysmal bone cyst is always secondary to some other primary process, although the original primary process may be obliterated by the presence and expansion of the aneurysmal cyst. Therefore, the wall of the cyst should be closely examined for evidence of a preexistent lesion.

REFERENCES

1. Kransdorf MJ, Moser RP Jr, Gilkey FW: Fibrous dysplasia (Review). *Radiographics* 10(3):519–537, 1990.
2. Ishida T, Dorfman HD: Massive chondroid differentiation in fibrous dysplasia of bone (fibrocartilaginous dysplasia). *Am J Surg Pathol* 17(9):924–930, 1993.
3. Arata MA, Peterson HA, Dahlin DC: Pathologic fractures through non-ossifying fibromas. *J Bone Joint Surg* 63A: 1177–1188, 1987.
4. Desprechins B, Freson M, De Boeck H, et al: Ossifying fibroma of the long bones. Radiologic diagnosis, differential diagnosis and management implications. *J Belge Radiol* 74(2):121–124, 1991.
5. Park YK, Unni KK, McLeod RA, et al: DJ: Osteofibrous dysplasia: Clinicopathologic study of 80 cases. *Hum Pathol* 24(12):1339–1347, 1993.
6. Alguacil-Garcia A, Alonso A, Pettigrew N: Osteofibrous dysplasia (ossifying fibroma) of the tibia and fibula and adamantinoma. *Am J Clin Pathol* 82:470–474, 1984.
7. Markel SF: Ossifying fibroma of long bone. *Am J Clin Pathol* 69:91–97, 1978.
8. Sweet DE, Vinh TN, Devaney K: Cortical osteofibrous dysplasia of long bone and its relationship to adamantinoma. A clinicopathologic study of 30 cases. *Am J Surg Pathol* 16(3):282–290, 1992.
9. Ueda Y, Roessner A, Bosse A, et al: Juvenile intracortical adamantinoma of the tibia with predominant osteofibrous dysplasia-like features (Review). *Pathol Res Pract* 187(8): 1039–1043; discussion 1043–1044, 1991.
10. Springfield DS, Rosenber AE, Mankin HJ, et al: Relationship between osteofibrous dysplasia and adamantinoma. *Clin Orth Res* 309:234–244, 1994.
11. Gebhardt MC, Campbell CJ, Schiller AL, et al: Desmoplastic fibroma of bone. *J Bone Joint Surg* 67(A):732–747, 1985.
12. Inwards CY, Unni KK, Beabout JW, et al: Desmoplastic fibroma of bone. *Cancer* 68(9):1978–1983, 1991.
13. Capanna R, Bertoni F, Bacchini P, et al: Malignant fibrous histiocytoma of bone. The experience at the Rizzoli Institute. Report of 90 cases. *Cancer* 54:177–187, 1984.
14. Johnson L: Personal communication. Armed Forces Institute of Pathology, Orthopedic Branch.
15. Campanacci M, Capanna R, Picci P: Unicameral and aneurysmal bone cysts. *Clin Orthop* 204:25–35, 1986.
16. Vergel De Dios AM, Bond JR, Shives TC, et al: Aneurysmal bone cyst. A clinicopathologic study of 238 cases. *Cancer* 69(12):2921–2931, 1992.
17. Bertoni F, Bacchini P, Capanna R, et al: Solid variant of aneurysmal bone cyst. *Cancer* 71(3):729–734, 1993.

6

Giant Cell Tumor of Bone

At the growth plate, osteoclasts are found on the metaphyseal side, removing the calcified cartilage matrix and eroding the chondrocytic lacunar space, allowing vascular invasion of cartilage. In addition to the erosion of the calcified cartilage, the osteoclasts also remove the primary trabeculae of bone in conjunction with the remodeling process. Based on this normal skeletal development the osteoclast is a metaphyseal cell, with a tendency to grow toward the epiphysis. It is therefore not surprising that the giant cell tumor of bone originates in the metaphysis, but after closure of the growth plate always involves the epiphysis as well. As opposed to the chondroblastoma, whose epicenter is always in the epiphyseal portion of the bone, the epicenter of the giant cell tumor is always beneath the growth plate on the metaphyseal portion of the bone. The defect is lytic, with sharply circumscribed margins. There may be expansion of the cortex and the lesion may actually break out of the bone. There is usually no discernible radiographic ossification. There may be reinforcement of remaining trabeculae to support the structure of bone, so a "soap bubble" pattern is seen in older lesions, whereas early lesions are simply lytic defects. Evidence of periosteal reaction such as sunburst, onion peel, or Codman triangle is not consistent with the diagnosis of giant cell tumor and suggests either a malignant process or secondary aneurysmal bone cyst formation (Figures 6-1, 6-2).[1–6]

The histology consists of giant cells and stromal cells. The stromal cell nucleus is identical to that of the giant cell. The giant cells may achieve large size with up to 100 nuclei in the older cells. Occasional minute foci of osteoid are not uncommon in giant cell tumor, but the lesion never contains cartilage. Occasional areas exhibit a fibrous pattern. The basic pattern of giant cells and identical stromal cells must be present to establish the diagnosis. The pleomorphism and mitotic activity occasionally seen in the stromal cells had led to grading of giant cell tumors. However, there is no demonstrable benefit, and it has no relationship to malignancy or aggressive behavior.

Extension into soft tissue or into vessels is not uncommon and does not signify malignancy. Most so-called malignant giant cell tumors of bone represent a *de novo* sarcoma coexisting with giant cells. These tumors often occur after radiation of a benign giant cell tumor, or coexisted as a malignant fibrosarcoma or osteosarcoma from the very beginning.

Occasional metastases from a giant cell tumor may appear in the lung.[7–9] These lesions follow surgery, may regress spontaneously and should be observed for evidence of aggressive growth prior to pulmonary surgery. "Cherry picking" surgery in these cases has been successful.

Numerous lesions of bone exhibit focal areas with numerous giant cells, especially chondroblastoma, but also nonossifying fibroma, osteoblastoma, osteosarcoma, and the aneurysmal bone cyst. These lesion may also present focal areas in which giant cells predominate. The diagnosis of giant cell tumor depends upon the identical nucleus of the stromal cell and the giant cell. The radiographic appearance should help establish the correct diagnosis.

Additional lesions in the differential diagnosis include the giant cell tumor of tendon sheath. These lesions have a propensity to invade the adjacent bone, and may then present diagnostic difficulties. A giant cell tumor of tendon sheath, even when invading bone, contains a varied stromal component, including numerous xanthoma cells, fibrous connective tissue elements, collagen fiber formation, hemosiderin, and foam-laden macrophages (Figures 6-3 to 6-17).

DIFFERENTIAL DIAGNOSIS OF LESIONS WITH NUMEROUS GIANT CELLS

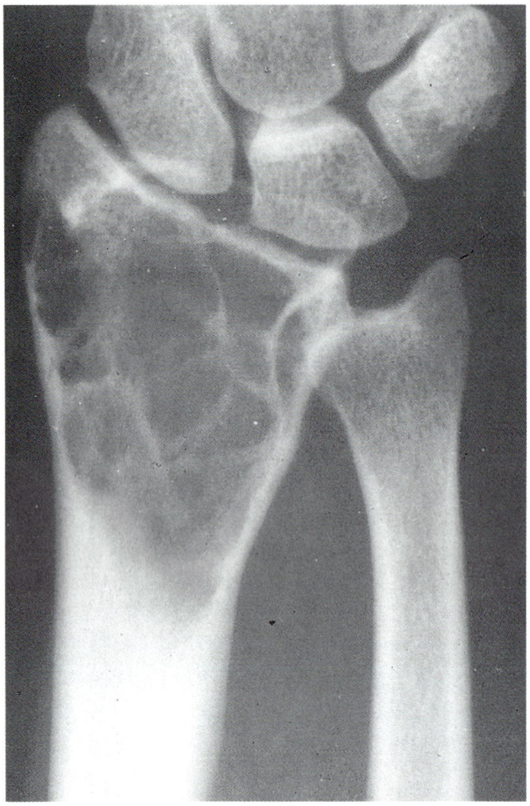

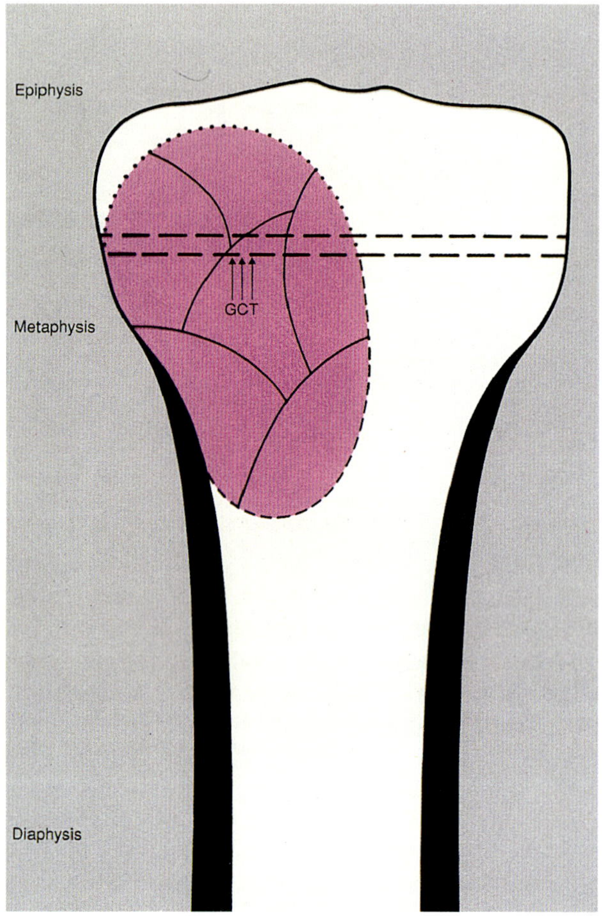

Figures 6-1, 6-2. The osteoclasts normally inhabit the metaphyseal portion of the growth plate, where they help to remodel the bone structure as it is formed. Therefore, the giant cell tumor of bone, of osteoclastic derivation, is usually metaphyseal when it originates, but tends to grow upward and involve the epiphysis at an early age. These lesions are large, usually eccentric, sharply circumscribed, may expand the bone somewhat, may have secondary aneurysmal bone cyst, but are usually benign. They may extend into soft tissue. Their characteristics are more aggressive than the other benign lesions of bone, and pulmonary implants are sometimes associated with giant cell tumors of bone. The characteristic septation within the older giant cell tumor indicates its slow-growing benign nature.

DIFFERENTIAL DIAGNOSIS OF LESIONS WITH NUMEROUS GIANT CELLS

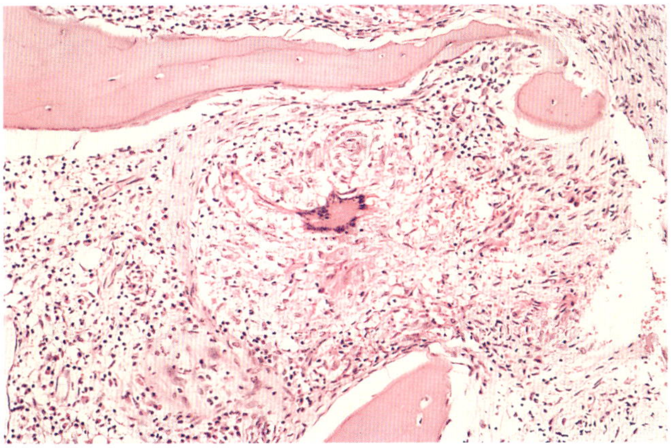

Figure 6-3. Granulomatous disease of bone. A sharply circumscribed granuloma, with a Langhans type giant cell in the center of the lesion between trabeculae of bone. Note the central area of histiocytic proliferation surrounded by a fibrous capsule, in turn surrounded by chronic inflammatory cells.

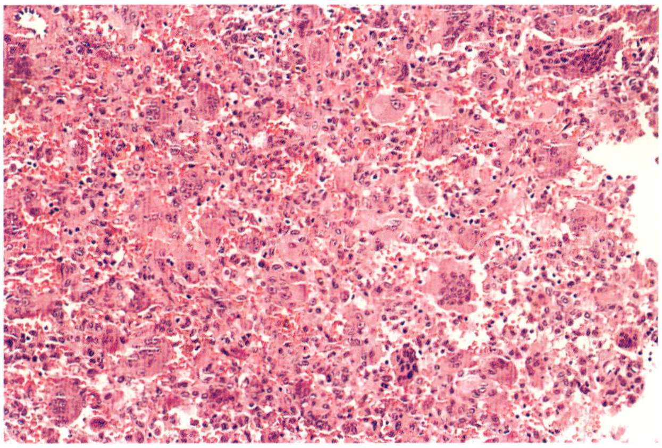

Figure 6-4. Giant cell tumor of bone. Note the uniform nuclear characteristics of the giant cell and the stromal cell and the interchangeability of both.

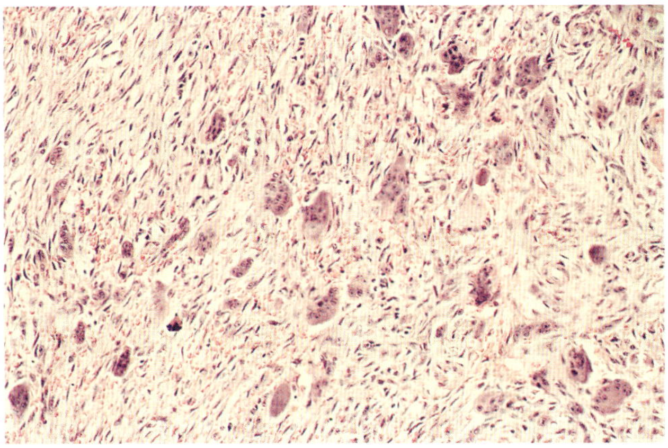

Figure 6-5. Brown tumor of hyperparathyroidism. Note numerous giant cells and a spindled connective tissue stroma.

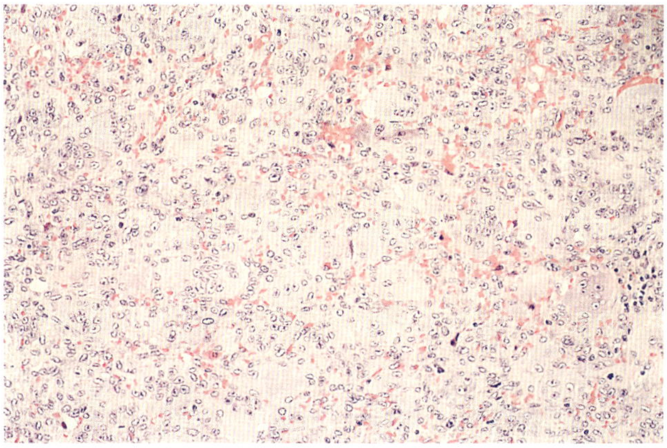

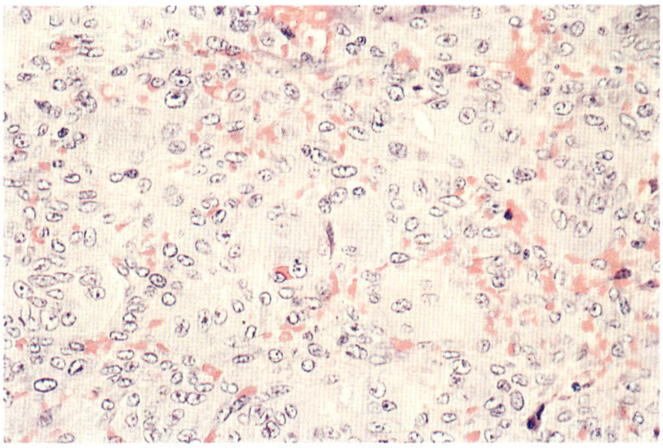

Figures 6-6, 6-7. Giant cell tumor in which the multinucleated giant cell is virtually indistinguishable for the stromal cell. The nuclei are identical, and can be interchanged with any of the nuclei within the giant cell.

DIFFERENTIAL DIAGNOSIS OF LESIONS WITH NUMEROUS GIANT CELLS

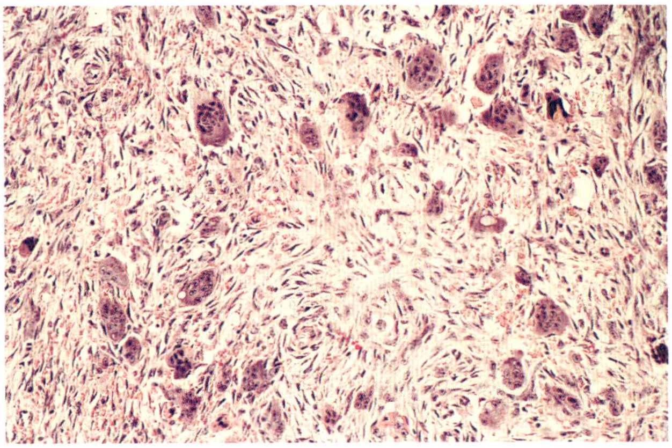

Figure 6-8. Brown tumor of hyperparathyroidism. Numerous giant cells accompanied by a spindle-shaped stroma. The presence of numerous spindled cells is not consistent with a bona fide giant cell tumor of bone.

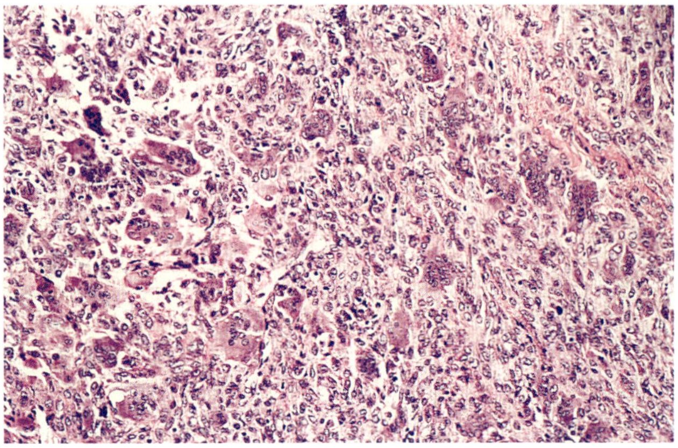

Figure 6-9. Giant cell reparative granuloma. Numerous giant cells, a markedly varied stromal component including numerous inflammatory cells. These lesions are usually confined to the jaw bones or to the distal appendages.

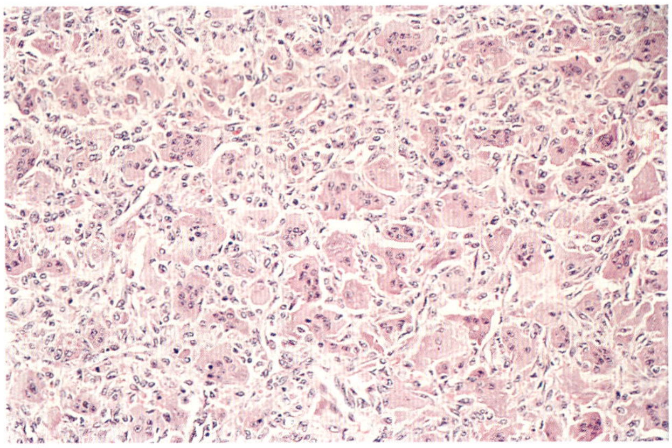

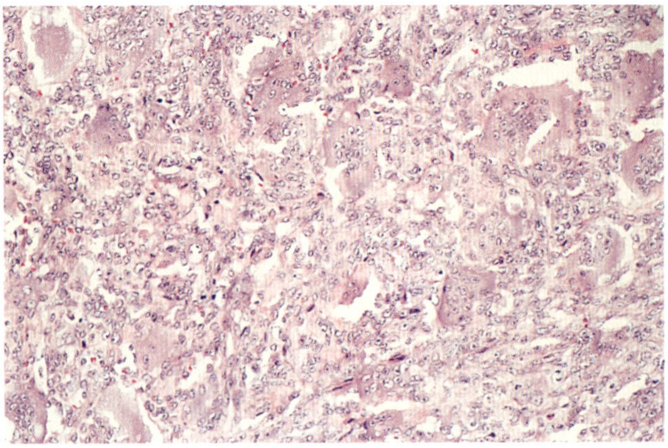

Figures 6-10, 6-11. Giant cell tumor of bone. Note the uniform nuclear characteristics of the giant cell and the stromal cell and the interchangeability of both.

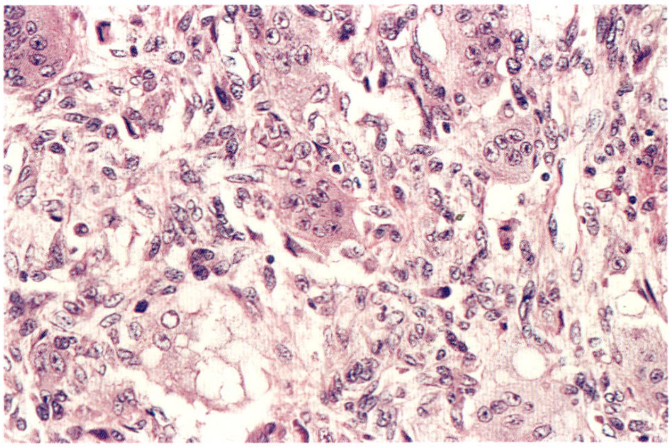

Figure 6-12. Giant cell reparative granuloma. Giant cell, with typical nucleus of the giant cell, stromal cells exhibiting moderate variability, but accompanied by fibrous connective tissue, xanthomatous elements and inflammatory elements.

DIFFERENTIAL DIAGNOSIS OF LESIONS WITH NUMEROUS GIANT CELLS

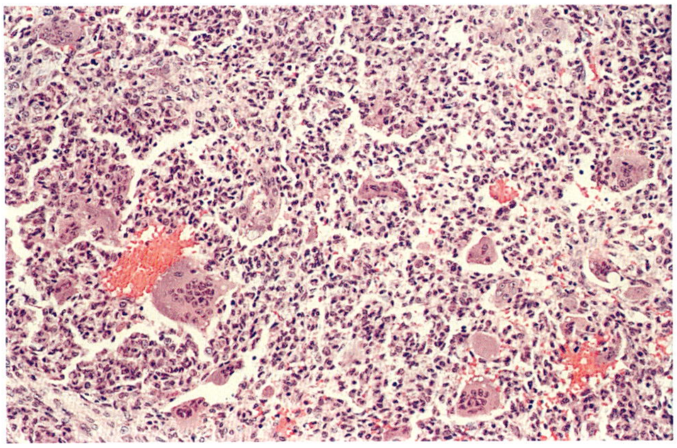

Figure 6-13. Chondroblastoma with numerous giant cells. In a field of this nature it is difficult to differentiate the bona fide giant cell tumor of bone from the chondroblastoma. A chondroblastoma must exhibit focal areas of calcification, cartilage formation, and the stromal cell tends to have more definable cytologic margins than the stromal cell of the giant cell tumor.

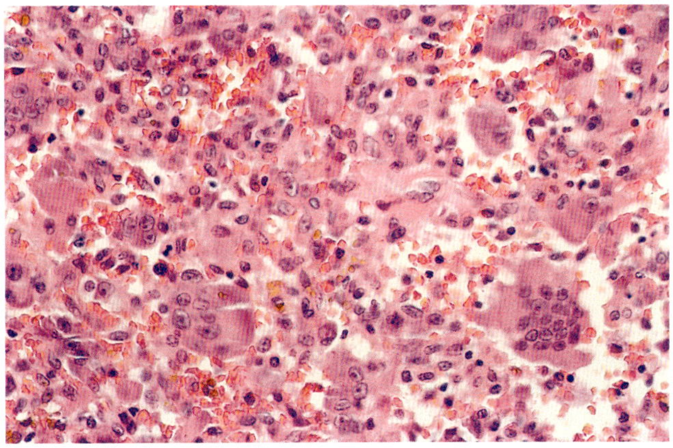

Figure 6-14. Giant cell tumor of bone. As opposed to the chondroblastoma, the stromal cells tend to blend with one another without distinct cytologic margins.

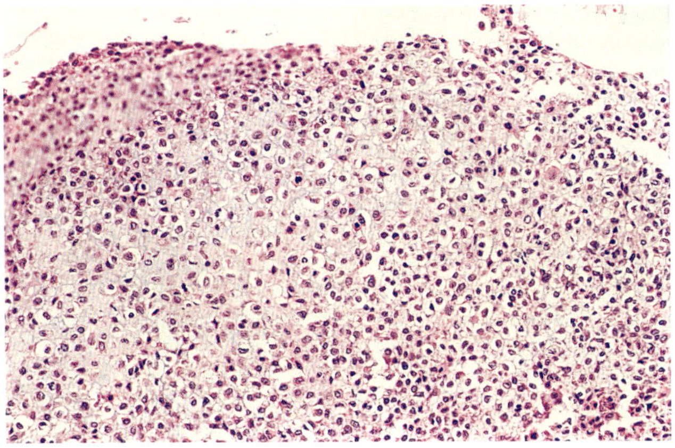

Figure 6-15. Chondroblastoma. Identifiable areas of cartilage are present in this chondroblastoma, but may be very discrete. Cartilage differentiation should never be present in a giant cell tumor of bone. Osteoid formation should not be present in a chondroblastoma.

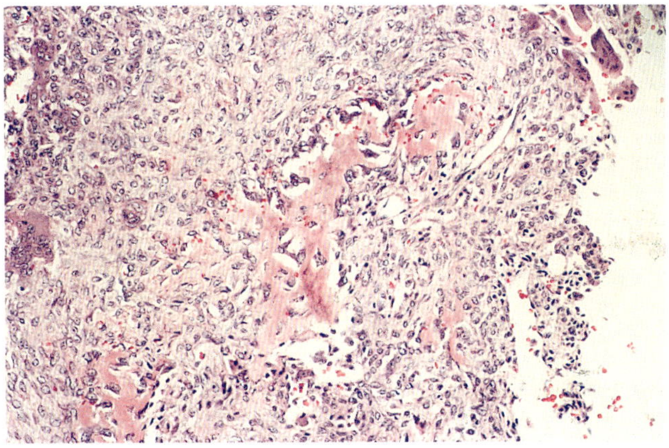

Figure 6-16. Focal areas of bone formation within a giant cell tumor. The giant cell tumor may form isolated small islands of osteoid.

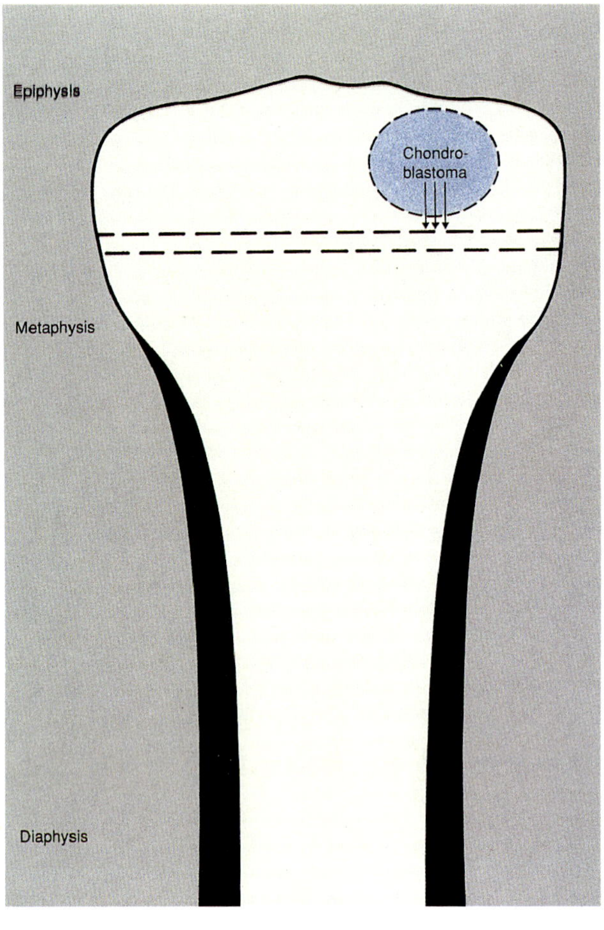

Figure 6-17. As opposed to the giant cell tumor of bone, the chondroblastoma is always epiphyseal in location, and may extend into the metaphysis only when the growth plate fuses. Thus, chondroblastomas have their epicenter within the epiphysis; giant cell tumors in the metaphysis.

MANAGEMENT OF GIANT CELL TUMOR

Because the bona fide giant cell tumor of bone frequently involves a young individual in the second or third decade of life, management of lesions about the knee pose serious difficulties. Resection, to include the joint, results in prosthesis at an early age, with attendant difficulties in later life. On the other hand, the tendency for local recurrence has led to an aggressive approach, including wide resection. While it is not the purpose of this text to recommend specific therapy, one should remember that the giant cell tumor of bone is a benign lesion despite the occasional pulmonary implants. An attempt at curettement with postoperative sterilization of the cavity would seem to be a reasonable approach, at least at first try, when either the femur or tibia is involved.[10–12] Segmental resection of bone is perfectly appropriate when dealing with giant cell tumors of radius or ulna, but in the experience of individuals treating giant cell tumors of bone, an attempt at either phenolization, cryosurgery, or other methods of cavity sterilization seems appropriate, at least on the first try.[13] Simple curettage without any effort to sterilize the resultant cavity is associated with a high and basically unacceptable recurrence rate.

GIANT CELL REPARATIVE GRANULOMA OF BONE

The giant cell reparative granuloma is a lesion which has been confused with the bona fide giant cell tumor.[14] It is predominantly found in the maxillary and mandibular bones, but can be found in the small bones of the hand, as well as other locations. The lesion is a benign reactive process which responds well to simple excision, i.e., curettage.[15]

The characteristic histologic features of the giant cell reparative granuloma include a highly cellular mass with numerous giant cells, an inflammatory component replacing the stromal component, hemorrhage, and some reactive bone formation. This lesion is common in the oral pathology literature, but when it involves bones other than jaw bones, the differential diagnosis between a giant cell reparative granuloma[14] and a bona fide giant cell tumor of bone may be difficult (Figures 6-9 to 6-12).

REFERENCES

1. Campanacci M, Baldini N, Boriani S, et al: Giant cell tumor of bone. *J Bone Joint Surg* 69A:106–114, 1987.
2. Carrasco CH, Murray JA: Giant cell tumors. *Ortho Clin North America* 30:395–405, 1989.
3. Komiya S, Inoue A: Cementation in the treatment of giant cell tumor of bone. *Arch Orthop Trauma Surg* 112(2): 51–55, 1993.
4. Kransdorf MJ, Sweet DE, Buetow PC. et al: Giant cell tumor in skeletally immature patients. *Radiology* 184(1): 233–237, 1992.
5. Manaster BJ, Doyle AJ: Giant cell tumors of bone (Review). *Radiol Clin North Am* 31(2):299–323, 1993.
6. Wold LE, Spelsberg T, Jiang N, et al: Steroid receptors and giant cell tumor of bone. *Current Topics in Pathology* 80:153–164, 1989.

7. Bertoni F, Present D, Sudanese A, et al: Giant-cell tumor of bone with pulmonary metastases. Six case reports and a review of the literature. *Clin Orthop Rel Res* 237:275–285, 1988.
8. Maloney WJ, Vaughan LM, Jones HH, et al: Benign metastasizing giant-cell tumor of bone. Report of three cases and review of the literature. *Clin Orthop Rel Res* 243: 208–215, 1989.
9. Tubbs WS, Brown LR, Beabout JW, et al: Benign giant-cell tumor of bone with pulmonary metastases: Clinical findings and radiologic appearance of metastases in 13 cases. *Am J Roentgenol* 158(2):331–334, 1992.
10. Pals SD, Wilkins RM: Giant cell tumor of bone treated by curettage, cementation, and bone grafting. *Orthopedics* 15(6):703–708, 1992.
11. Moser RP Jr, Kransdorf MJ, Gilkey FW, et al: From the archives of the AFIP. Giant cell tumor of the upper extremity. *Radiographics* 10(1):83–102, 1990.
12. Rooney RJ, Asirvatham R, Lifeso RM, et al: Giant cell tumour of bone. A surgical approach to grade III tumours. *Int Orthop* 17(2):87–92, 1993.
13. Vander Griend RA, Funderburk CH: The treatment of giant-cell tumors of the distal part of the radius. *J Bone Joint Surg Am* 75(6):899–908, 1993.
14. Oda Y, Tsuneyoshi M, Shinohara N: "Solid" variant of aneurysmal bone cyst (extragnathic giant cell reparative granuloma) in the axial skeleton and long bones. A study of its morphologic spectrum and distinction from allied giant cell lesions. *Cancer* 70(11):2642–2649, 1992.
15. Ratner V, Dorfman HD: Giant-cell reparative granuloma of the hand and foot bones. *Clin Orthop* 260:251–258, 1990.

7

Round Cell Lesions

Round cell lesions of bone are either monomorphous and polymorphous. The monomorphous form consists of an infiltrate with a single cell type. The cells vary in size, configuration, and nuclear chromatin pattern, but are all basically the same cell. A polymorphous infiltrate consists of more than one cell type, all clearly distinguishable. Eosinophilic granuloma of bone is an example of a polymorphous infiltrate, consisting of histiocytes, eosinophils, and numerous other inflammatory cells. Ewing's sarcoma is a monomorphous infiltrate. The first task of the pathologist is to determine whether the round cell infiltrate is mono- or polymorphous. The differential diagnosis of the polymorphous infiltrates includes osteomyelitis, eosinophilic granuloma, inflammatory or reactive processes of any kind, and also skeletal involvement in Hodgkin's disease. The differential diagnosis of the various monomorphous infiltrates is listed in Table 7-1.

Whenever one considers small cell neoplasms of bone one must obviously include the possibility of metastatic small cell osteosarcoma[1] or small cell carcinoma. Usually the immunohistochemical characteristics of the small cell metastatic carcinoma serve to differentiate it from the primary small cell tumors of bone, although at times the differential between mesenchymal chondrosarcoma, primary lymphoma, or small cell osteosarcoma can be exceedingly difficult. Whenever one is confronted with the differential diagnosis of these entities one must collect specimens for immunohistochemistry, electron microscopy, cytogenetic analysis, and sufficient tissue for careful histologic analysis. One should not forget that occasionally osteomyelitis may present with a sheet-like infiltrate of inflammatory cells, particularly plasma cells. Every biopsy requires a culture, and every culture requires a biopsy! (Figures 7-1 to 7-6).

EWING'S SARCOMA

Current concepts of Ewing's sarcoma indicate that the lesion is a primitive undifferentiated tumor of neuroectodermal origin, sharing some immunohistochemical characteristics with other primitive neuroectodermal tumors. Neuron-specific enolase, as well as glycogen production are the two immunohistochemical and histochemical features respectively which tend to confirm the presence of Ewing's sarcoma, as opposed to the other round cell tumors. In addition to these immunochemical and histochemical features, characteristic translocation of chromosomal material has been identified in the presence of Ewing's sarcoma. These translocations are not invariably present, but have been identified in approximately 85% of cases.[2–8]

The characteristic radiographic appearance of Ewing's sarcoma is permeative destruction, extensive periosteal reaction, and no evidence of calcifiable matrix formation. The radiographic differential diagnosis must always include the possibility of osteomyelitis. In addition, there are a variety of radiographic patterns that are associated with Ewing's sarcoma, including extensive sclerosis of the host bone as a reaction to the tumor. The tumor is quick to expand into the adjacent soft tissue and may actually appear to be periosteal in origin.[9,10]

The characteristic histologic pattern is a monomorphous round cell tumor, the nuclei are uniform in size,

TABLE 7-1. Small Cell Neoplasms of Bone

	*Ewing's**	*Metastatic Neuroblastoma*	*Primary Lymphoma*	*Small Cell Osteosarcoma*	*Mesenchymal Chondrosarcoma*
Peak age	2nd decade	< 5 years	broad	broad	broad
Male/female	1.5:1	equal	1.5:1	equal	equal
Bones favored	tubular	skull	tubular	tubular	flat
Extra-osseous mass	most	few	common	< 50%	common
Nuclear shape	oval to round	oval to round	variable, multilobulated	oval to spindled	oval to spindled
Multinucleated neoplastic cells	very rare*	occasional	common	± rare	± rare
True rosettes	absent	±10%	absent	absent	absent
Neuritic type extensions	absent	common	absent	absent	absent
Glycogen	prominent 75%, rare 10%	rare	absent	± present	rare

Adapted from Fechner RE: Workshop, ASCP, 1985.
*Excludes large cell variant.

and cytoplasmic boundaries are usually indistinct. There is great variety of this pattern, and occasionally oval shaped cells, elongated cells, pseudorosettes, filigree pattern, and even a lobular pattern may be seen. The significance of all these different histologic patterns is under debate; at least some of them appear to be associated with prognosis (Figures 7-7, 7-8).

The most readily useful diagnostic feature of Ewing's sarcoma is the presence of glycogen granules, which can be confirmed with periodic acid-Schiff (PAS) stains or electron microscopy. Embryonal rhabdomyosarcomas may also contain glycogen; however, the presence of glycogen helps to differentiate the tumor from neuroblastoma and malignant lymphoma.

Combined radiation and chemotherapy has significantly improved the prognosis for Ewing's sarcoma, which, prior to combined therapy, was almost a uniformly fatal disease. Current success rate is better than 50% survival although tumor location may affect survival.[11–18]

PERIPHERAL NEUROECTODERMAL TUMOR

In recent years it has become apparent that there are great similarities between the peripheral neuroectodermal tumor of childhood, a soft tissue sarcoma, and Ewing's sarcoma. They share a translocation chromosome, which can be identified in most of the cases of Ewing's sarcoma and peripheral neuroectodermal tumor. Although there are many similarities between the two entities, the ultrastructural analysis does allow for some differentiation between the two, and the peripheral neuroectodermal tumor does appear to be more aggressive. One must await further research on this subject which may well have important implications for treatment.[19,20]

PRIMARY LYMPHOMA OF BONE

The primary lymphoma of bone was formerly referred to as reticulum cell sarcoma of bone. Since the advent of histologic typing, it has been shown that most of these tumors are characteristic B or T cell lymphomas, confined to a single bone in the skeleton, at least at the time of first discovery. It is generally accepted that a lesion cannot be considered a primary lymphoma of bone if there is involvement of other sites, either prior to or immediately after the lesion is first discovered in the skeleton.[21]

The tumor behaves similarly to the other round cell neoplasms of bone, i.e., rapid destruction of both cortical and trabecular bone, and extension beyond the geographic confines of the skeletal structure into the adjacent soft tissue. A rather common feature of lymphoma is the widespread destruction of the bone and adjacent soft tissue with little if any radiographic evidence of this

ROUND CELL LESIONS OF THE SKELETON

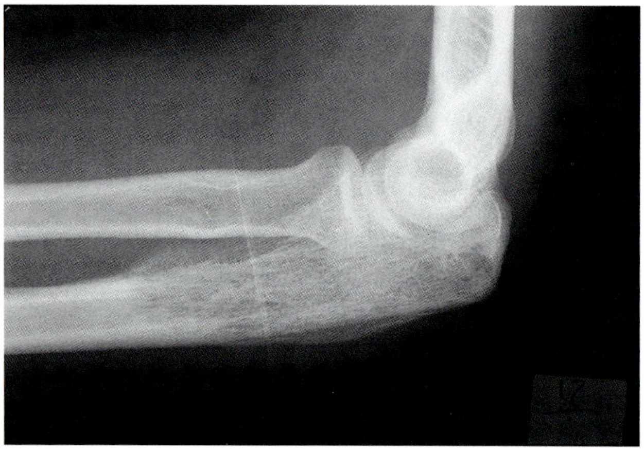

Figure 7-1. Round cell tumor of bone. Lytic destructive pattern in proximal portion of ulna, with periosteal reaction. Rapid permeative growth of the neoplastic process through the epiphysis and metaphysis of the ulna. No discerniable matrix production by the neoplastic process. There are no diagnostic features in this radiograph, except the assurance that one is dealing with a rapidly growing process, probably neoplastic.

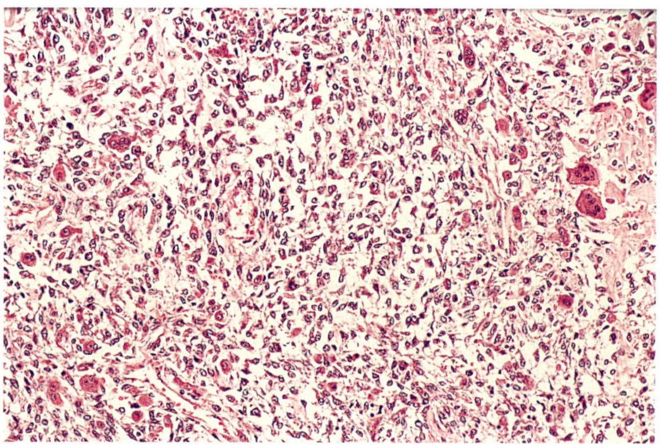

Figure 7-3. Small cell osteosarcoma. The lesion is difficult to diagnose without the presence of identifiable osteoid. In this illustration there are large numbers of proliferating small cells and occasional giant cells.

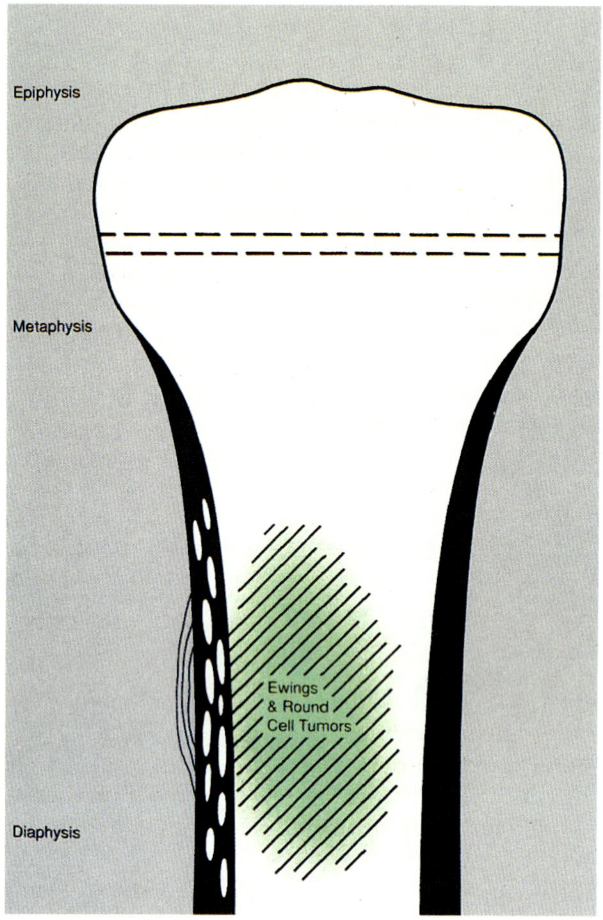

Figure 7-2. Classical features of a round cell tumor, consisting of a permeative pattern of destruction within cortex and trabecular bone, indistinct margins, usually an onion-peel type of periosteal reaction.

The radiographic manifestations of all round cell tumors are those of a rapidly growing process, permeative in nature, with poorly defined margins. Permeative destruction of the adjacent cortex is usually associated with round cell tumors, and periosteal reaction such as onion-peel or hair-on-end is a common associated feature. Although Ewing's sarcoma and lymphoma of bone may elicit a response on the part of the host, the tumor itself does not form any identifiable matrix.

ROUND CELL LESIONS OF THE SKELETON

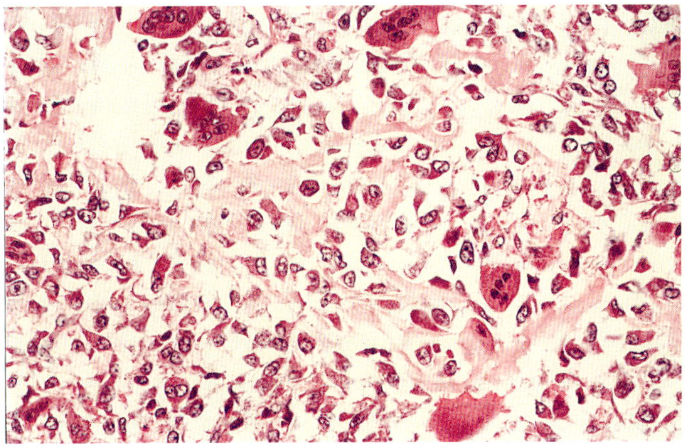

Figure 7-4. Small cell osteosarcoma. Distinct and identifiable osteoid formation by the tumor has to be searched for, and is often discrete.

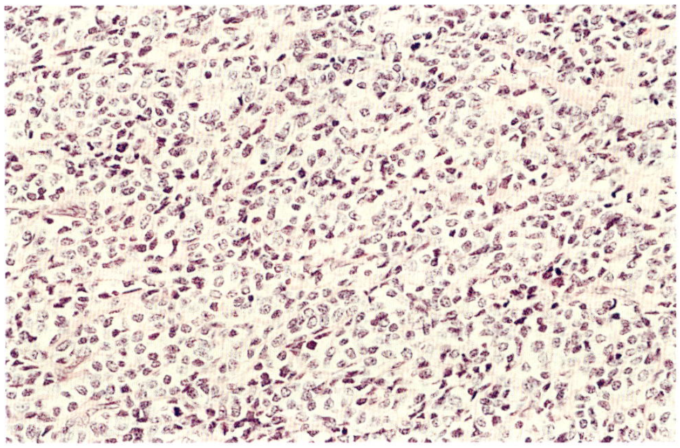

Figure 7-5. Mesenchymal chondrosarcoma. Note the uniform appearance of small cells, without significant pleomorphism.

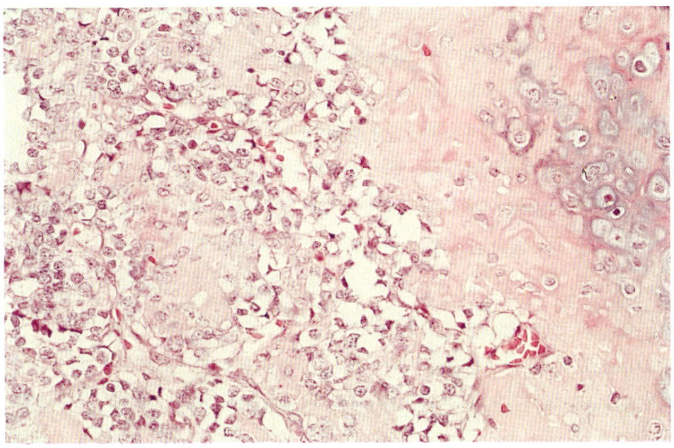

Figure 7-6. Mesenchymal chondrosarcoma. Isolated islands of identifiable cartilage in mesenchymal chondrosarcoma establish the diagnosis.

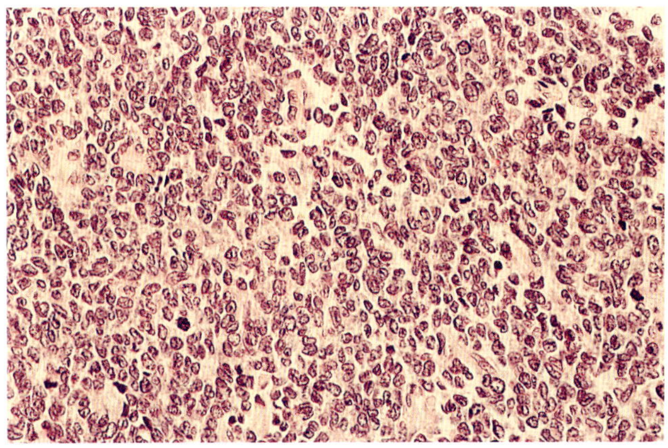

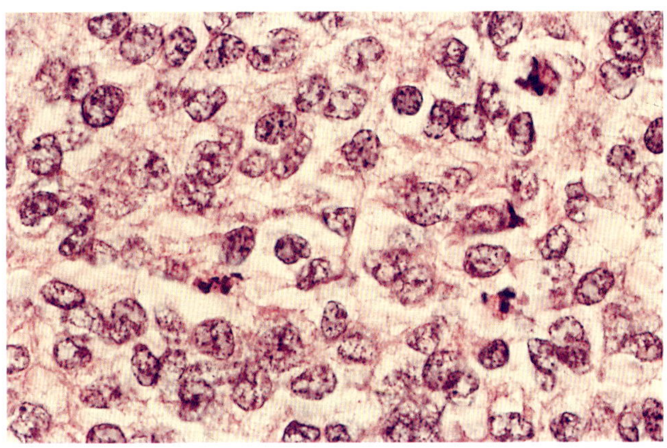

Figures 7-7, 7-8. Ewing's sarcoma. A sheet-like infiltrate of nuclei, without significant cytoplasmic content. Additional studies, such as determination of glycogen content by PAS stain or electron microscopy, are necessary to identify this tumor as a Ewing's sarcoma.

destructive process (Figure 7-9). The lesion is then discovered through a pathologic fracture or soft tissue mass.

As a rule, the primary lymphoma of bone involves an older age group than the patients with Ewing's sarcoma, but again, age and location within the skeleton are only adjunct criteria and not diagnostic. Diagnosis is established by the histologic features of the neoplasm: usually diffuse rather than nodular, monophasic B or T cells, and a tendency to a greater degree of pleomorphism, and more cytoplasmic differentiation than the typical Ewing's sarcoma. Lymphomas of bone do not contain glycogen.

ROUND CELL LESIONS OF THE SKELETON

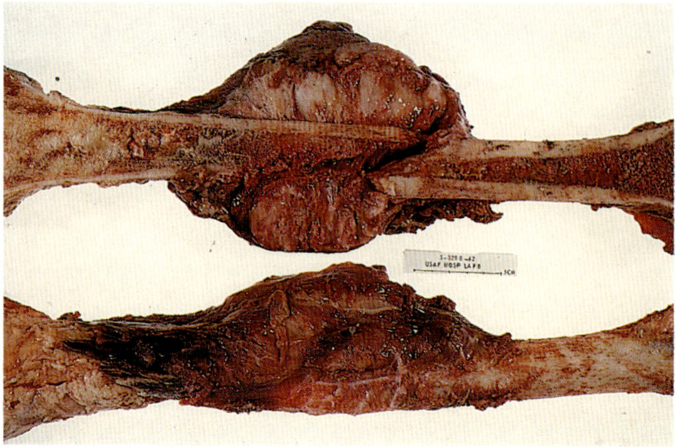

Figure 7-9. Primary lymphoma of bone. Extensive destruction and spread into soft tissue, with minimal damage to the bone itself.

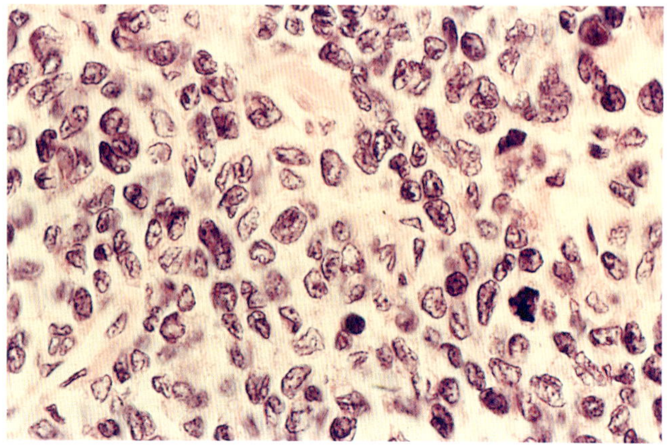

Figure 7-10. Primary lymphoma of bone. Cellular pleomorphism of primary lymphoma of bone is usually more extensive than in Ewing's sarcoma. Immunohistochemical typing of the round cell population is mandatory for diagnosis.

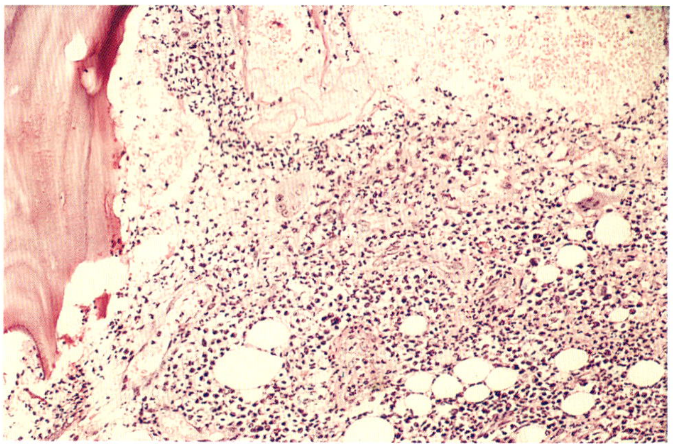

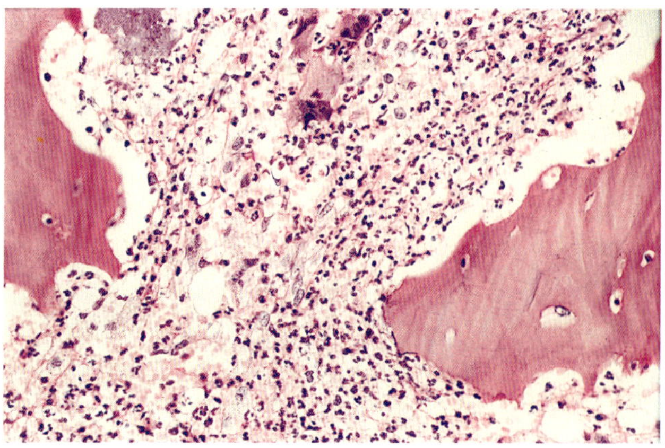

Figures 7-11, 7-12. Osteomyelitis. Replacement of normal hematopoietic tissue by a mixed cellular infiltrate, with Howship lacunae exhibiting destruction of cortical or trabecular bone. The cellular infiltrate is polymorphous.

As therapy is radically different from the other round cell tumors, an early and thorough effort should be made to differentiate the lymphoma of bone from the other round cell neoplasms. Histologic differentiation may be difficult, and immunohistochemistry, electron microscopy, and chromosomal markers may all have to be used to establish a definite differential diagnosis versus Ewing's sarcoma. It is therefore important for the pathologist to collect specimens for all of these studies, whenever confronted with a round cell tumor of bone (Figures 7-9, 7-10).

MULTIPLE MYELOMA

Multiple myeloma of bone is the most common primary neoplasm of bone. It may present in a variety of patterns: either as a single lytic lesion, or as multiple punched-out lytic lesions throughout the skeleton. Approximately 20% of patients with myeloma will not present with multiple lesions, but rather with diffuse osteoporosis of the skeleton.[22]

The plasma cell is a normal constituent of the hematopoietic tissue. As a result there appears to be no reaction to a neoplasm of plasma cells on the part of the host bone. There is therefore no reaction to the infiltration by the plasma cells, and the bone scan remains completely negative. Radiographic analysis will reveal punched-out lesions without evidence of a sclerotic reaction to the lytic process.

ROUND CELL LESIONS OF THE SKELETON

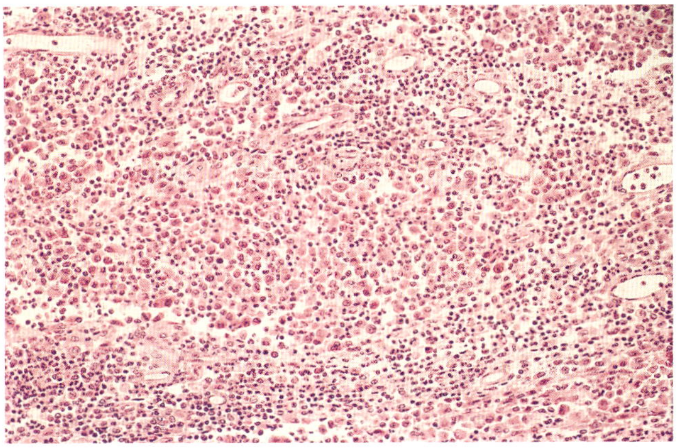

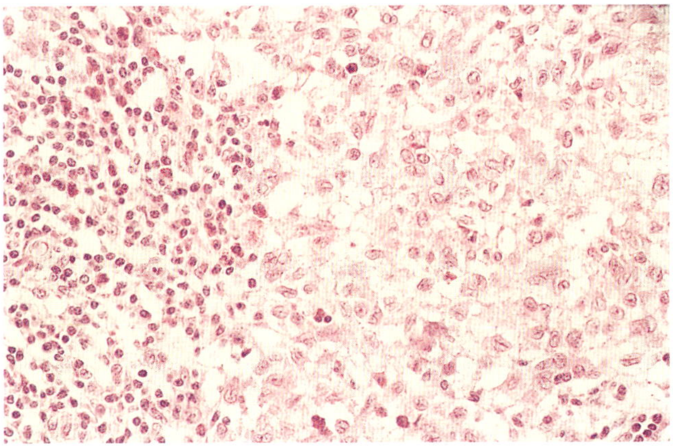

Figures 7-13, 7-14. Langerhans cell granuloma. A polymorphous infiltrate, including the large histiocyte, numerous smaller granulocytes, among them discernible eosinophilic granulocytes.

It is occasionally difficult to discriminate between the Langerhans cell granuloma and an osteomyelitis. If the issue cannot be resolved with histologic examination, electron microscopic examination would be required to demonstrate the Bierbeck granule in the Langerhans cell.

The diagnosis requires confirmation by the characteristic abnormalities in the serum protein, or, in the early cases, characteristic monoclonal abnormalities in urinary protein excretion. The differential diagnosis includes the small cell neoplasms of bone. Usually it is not difficult to differentiate a plasma cell neoplasm from Ewing's sarcoma, lymphoma, or the other small cell neoplasms; but occasionally immature plasma cells offer difficulties.

Of greater importance is to differentiate myeloma from a chronic inflammatory process within the bone. Plasma cell osteomyelitis may be seen in any chronic osteomyelitis, particularly *Salmonella* osteomyelitis. It results in a polymorphous infiltrate with numerous plasma cells, but also associated with a sclerotic reaction on the part of the host.

EOSINOPHILIC GRANULOMA OF BONE (LANGERHANS-CELL GRANULOMATOSIS)

This lesion is of uncertain etiology; the basic element is the Langerhans cell which contains the diagnostic Bierbeck granule. The cell is considered part of the monocyte-macrophage system, and although its precise function is unknown, it is related to cell-mediated immune reactions. The presence of this type of cell in numerous entities has led to the "histiocytosis X" designation.[23,24]

The typical eosinophilic granuloma is a sharply circumscribed lytic defect. The margins are sharp; there is some sclerosis although purely lytic defects are also common. Periosteal reactions may be present initially, but usually subside with modest expansion of cortex and reinforcement at the margin. The lesion tends to subside, which is reflected in the sharp margination, minimal sclerosis and ultimate healing of all eosinophilic granulomas. Vertebral involvement is relatively common, and may cause collapse, resulting in the characteristic vertebra plana.

The lesion is a *polymorphous* infiltrate, consisting of the characteristic Langerhans cell, granulocytes, particularly eosinophilic granulocytes, occasional lymphocytes and monocytes. The histologic appearance of eosinophilic granuloma of bone is indistinguishable from Hand-Schüller-Christian disease, and the clinical syndrome determines the appropriate name for the entity involved (Figures 7-11 to 7-14).

REFERENCES

1. Dickersin GR, Rosenberg AE: The ultrastructure of small-cell osteosarcoma, with a review of the light microscopy and differential diagnosis. *Hum Pathol* 22(3):267–275, 1991.
2. Ambros IM, Ambros PF, Strehl S, et al: MIC2 is a specific marker for Ewing's sarcoma and peripheral primitive neuroectodermal tumors. Evidence for a common histogenesis of Ewing's sarcoma and peripheral primitive neuroectodermal tumors from MIC2 expression and specific chromosome aberration. *Cancer* 67(7):1886–1893, 1991.
3. Donovan MJ, Hempsterad BL, Horvath C, et al: Immunohistochemical localization of Trk receptor protein in pediatric small round blue cell tumors. *Am J Pathol* 143(6): 1560–1567, 1993.

4. Downing JR, Head DR, Parham DM, et al: Detection of the (11;22) (q24;q12) translocation of Ewing's sarcoma and peripheral neuroectodermal tumor by reverse transcription polymerase chain reaction. *Am J Pathol* 143(5): 1294–1300, 1993.
5. Fellinger EJ, Garin-Chesa P, Triche TJ, et al: Immunohistochemical analysis of Ewing's sarcoma cell surface antigen p30/32MIC2. *Am J Pathol* 139(2):317–325, 1991.
6. Ladanyi M, Lewis R, Garin-Chesa P, et al: EWS rearrangement in Ewing's sarcoma and peripheral neuroectodermal tumor. Molecular detection and correlation with cytogenetic analysis and MIC2 expression. *Diagn Mol Pathol* 2(3):141–146, 1993.
7. Taylor C, Patel K, Jones T, et al: Diagnosis of Ewing's sarcoma and peripheral neuroectodermal tumour based on the detection of t(11;22) using fluorescence in situ hybridisation. *Br J Cancer* 67(1):128–133, 1993.
8. Navarro S, Cavazzana, Llombart-Bosch A, et al: Comparison of Ewing's sarcoma of bone and peripheral neuroepithelioma. *Arch Pathol Lab Med* 118:608–615, 1994.
9. Eggli KD, Quiogue T, Moser RP Jr: Ewing's sarcoma (Review). *Radiol Clin North Am* 31(2):325–337, 1993.
10. Wuisman P, Roessner A, Blasius S, et al: (Sub)periosteal Ewing's sarcoma of bone. *J Cancer Res Clin Oncol* 118(1): 72–74, 1992.
11. Barbieri E, Emiliani E, Zini G, et al: Combined therapy of localized Ewing's sarcoma of bone: Analysis of results of 100 patients. *Int J Radiat Oncol Biol Phys* 19(5):1165–1170, 1990.
12. Frassica FJ, Frassica DA, Pritchard DJ, et al: Ewing sarcoma of the pelvis. Clinicopathological features and treatment. *J Bone Joint Surg Am* 75(10):1457–1465, 1993.
13. Horowitz ME, Neff JR, Kun LE: Ewing's sarcoma. Radiotherapy versus surgery for local control (Review). *Pediatr Clin North Am* 38(2):365–380, 1991.
14. Jurgens H, Exner U, Gadner H, et al: Multidisciplinary treatment of primary Ewing's sarcoma of bone. A 6-year experience of a European Cooperative trail. *Cancer* 61: 23–32, 1988.
15. Kinsella TJ, Miser JS, Waller B, et al: Long-term follow-up of Ewing's sarcoma of bone treated with combined modality therapy. *Int J Radiat Oncol Biol Phys* 20(3):389–395, 1991.
16. O'Connor MI, Pritchard DJ: Ewing's sarcoma. Prognostic factors, disease control, and the reemerging role of surgical treatment (Review). *Clin Orthop* 262:78–87, 1991.
17. Toni A, Neff JR, Sudanese A, et al: The role of surgical therapy in patients with nonmetastatic Ewing's sarcoma of the limbs. *Clin Orthop* 286:225–240, 1993.
18. Toni A, Sudanese A, Ciaroni, et al: The role of surgery in the local treatment of Ewing's sarcoma of the extremities. *Chir Organi Mov* 75(Suppl 1):262–264, 1990.
19. Dehner LP: Neuroepithelioma (primitive neuroectodermal tumor) and Ewing's sarcoma. At least a partial consensus (Editorial). *Arch Pathol Lab Med* 118:606–607, 1994.
20. Schmidt D, Herrmann C, Jurgens H, et al: Malignant peripheral neuroectodermal tumor and its necessary distinction from Ewing's sarcoma. A report from the Kiel Pediatric Tumor Registry. *Cancer* 68(10):2251–2259, 1991.
21. Schajowicz F: *Tumors and Tumorlike Lesions of Bone. Pathology, Radiology, and Treatment.* Berlin, Springer-Verlag 1994, pp 328–341.
22. Kyle RA: Multiple myeloma, review of 869 cases. *Mayo Clinic Proc* 50:29–40, 1975.
23. Favara B, McCarthy R, Mierau G: Histiocytosis X. *Hum Pathol* 14:663–676, 1993.
24. Malkey JT, Carter JR: Eosinophilic granuloma of bone. *Clin Orthop* 204:37–44, 1986.

8

Synovial and Soft Tissue Lesions

SYNOVIAL LESIONS

The synovial surface is lined by two layers of cells: type A, a macrophage-like cell that phagocytoses, and type B, a fibroblast-like cell that produces multiple substances, including proteinase, collagenase, hyaluronic acid, and prostaglandins. Synovial fluid is a product of plasma plus the unique products of the synovial membrane. The synovial fluid is expressed by the synovium, and serves to provide nutriment to the cartilage. The phagocytic properties of the synovium serve to absorb synovial fluid with metabolic waste products of cartilage metabolism.

Cartilaginous Lesions

There are several cartilaginous lesions that may involve the joint capsule or synovium: primary synovial chondromatosis, secondary synovial chondrometaplasia, para-articular chondroma, para-articular osteochondroma, as well as chondromas of hands and feet extending into synovium.

Synovial chondromatosis and secondary synovial chondrometaplasia are similar, but may be divided into distinct groups on the basis of an intrasynovial chondrometaplasia without loose bodies, intrasynovial disease with loose bodies, and finally, bodies without synovial disease. True synovial chondromatosis is a metaplastic process involving the synovium, with metaplasia of synovial tissue to form mature cartilage. Because the blood supply of the synovium is maintained, there may well be bone formation, and in those instances the disease state is called synovial osteochondromatosis. There is no associated osteochondritis, and articular cartilage is uninvolved. Since the lesion involves the synovium, the only cure is total synovectomy.[1] Despite its somewhat ominous appearance, synovial chondromatosis should never be treated as a malignant process, and conservative therapy is appropriate. There are extremely isolated cases of malignant transformation;[2,3] on the whole, it is a safe assumption that malignant transformation of synovial chondromatosis will not occur.

Secondary synovial chondrometaplasia occurs when there is a defect in the articular cartilage, with resultant shedding of cartilaginous cells into the joint space, subsequent accretion of cartilage cells to the cartilaginous nidus, with the formation of numerous, partially calcified, cartilaginous masses. If the origin of this cartilaginous shedding is in the articular surface, occasional bone fragments are included in the material shed into the joint space. Since this shedding results in loss of blood supply, any bone that is associated with this shedding process is immediately infarcted and will appear as nonviable remnants of bone (and infarcted marrow). Cartilage receives all its nutrition from synovial fluid, continues to grow, and these "loose bodies" may therefore attain considerable size and calcify. A connective tissue membrane may surround these loose bodies and assume synovial characteristics. Under those conditions, the lesion is known as a secondary synovial chondromatosis.

A para-articular chondroma, or para-articular osteochondroma is simply a cartilaginous lesion arising in soft tissue. These lesions are benign chondromas of soft tissue origin, and simple excision is adequate and appropriate therapy.

Both synovial chondromatosis and the soft tissue chondromas may exhibit marked pleomorphism, hyperchromatic nuclei, cellular atypism, and even mitotic activity. They are not malignant lesions. The histologic appearance which would ordinarily be extremely worrisome in an intraskeletal site can be discounted both in the synovial chondromatosis and the para-articular chondromas (Figures 8-1 to 8-4).

Synovitis

Nodular synovitis and pigmented villonodular synovitis are basically variants of the same disease. Tenosynovial tissue, including tendon sheath, synovium and other articular structures, is capable of proliferating and forming nodular lesions. These are composed of mesenchymal derivatives, including fibroblasts, histiocytes, and myofibroblasts. Synovial cells are difficult to identify, since they have the same morphologic characteristics as the histiocytes.

Localized Nodular Synovitis (Table 8-1)

Localized nodular synovitis or giant cell tumor of tendon sheath is a localized nodule, usually yellow or yellow-brown in color. The yellow color is due to the xanthomatous component of the lesion. Numerous giant cells are present; hemosiderin pigmentation may be noted; fibroblasts, histiocytes, xanthoma cells and fairly pleomorphic mesenchymal cells also may be part of the lesion. The lesion may also invade bone and cause radiographically identifiable defects, especially in the small bones of the hands and feet.[4]

Pigmented Villonodular Synovitis (Table 8-1)

Pigmented villonodular form (diffuse), or the localized nodular form can vary in its clinical expression. The spectrum varies from an incidental finding at arthroscopy to the rather complicated and prolonged serious debilitating illness. From a histologic viewpoint, the lesion is characterized by the presence of numerous multinucleated giant cells, which are derived from the marrow monocyte/macrophage lineage.[5] The giant cells are accompanied by fibrous connective tissue, xanthomatous cells with numerous fat-laden macrophages, and variable degrees of hemosiderin deposition within the tissue. The capability to invade bone is shared by both the nodular and the diffuse form, so that one can demonstrate the nodular synovitis invading the bony component of small bones in the hands and feet, and at the same time, the diffuse pigmented form can and frequently does invade bone structures, particularly in the knee and hip.

Villonodular synovitis may be present in almost any joint of the human body and unusual sites often lead to difficulty in diagnosis (Figures 8-5 to 8-13).[6–8]

The differential diagnosis (Table 8-2) includes soft tissue proliferations, predominantly synovial chondromatosis, inflammatory diseases with synovial proliferation such as rheumatoid arthritis, a less common fibroma of tendon sheath,[9,10] and malignant soft tissue tumors. As a rule, soft tissue sarcomas do not involve the joint space itself, and villonodular synovitis, unless it arises in a bursa, is invariably associated with the synovial lining surface of a joint (Figures 8-14, 8-15).

Diagnosis is best established by biopsy. Radiographic studies demonstrate the presence of a soft tissue mass, but magnetic resonance imaging (MRI) studies are particularly helpful.[11–13] The hemosiderin deposition results in a loss of signal intensity, which the radiologist utilizes to suggest the diagnosis of pigmented villonodular synovitis as opposed to the other lesions. Aspiration of the joint fluid may exhibit the foam-laden macrophage with its characteristic Maltese cross,[14] and fine needle biopsy has also been used.[15] However, arthroscopic surgery appears to be the most frequent diagnostic tool utilized by the orthopaedic community.

The lesion may be aggressive. It often infiltrates into surrounding structures, surrounding nerves, vessels and into the bone itself. Indeed, multiple adjacent bones are often involved, which certainly helps to narrow the differential diagnosis into lesions of synovial, vascular, or inflammatory origin.

Simple surgical excision of the lesion is the recommended therapy. A recurrence rate of approximately 25% has been documented,[16,17] but even so, simple excision of the recurrent process is recommended. Radical procedures are not appropriate for this condition, despite the isolated case report of a malignant tumor (Figures 8-5 to 8-9).[18]

SOFT TISSUE SARCOMAS

There are numerous soft tissue sarcomas, including all forms of extraskeletal osteosarcomas and chondrosarco-

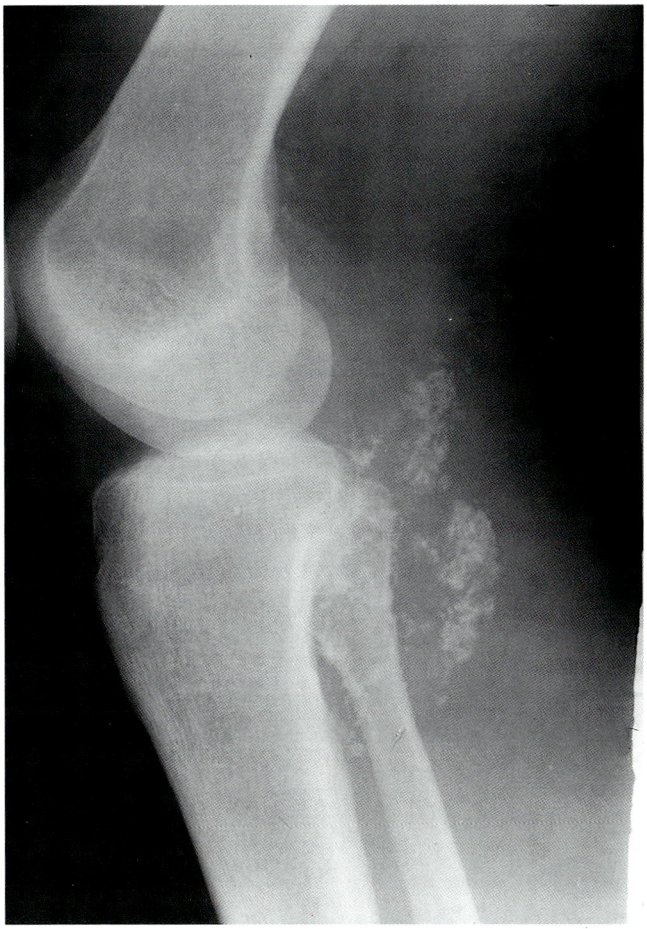

Figure 8-1. Radiograph of synovial chondromatosis. Note the calcified bodies within the joint space, but not within the bone. The pattern is flocculent, consistent with cartilage.

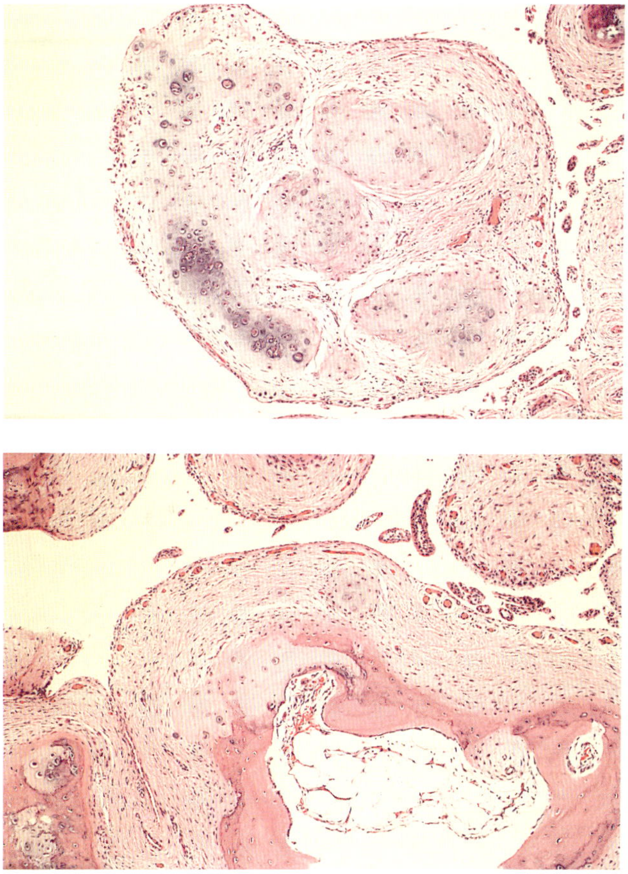

Figures 8-3, 8-4. Synovial chondromatosis tends to form nodules and lobular fragments of cartilage, surrounded by the synovial-type epithelium. Because the blood supply is maintained, the cartilage goes on to transform into bone and may contain normal marrow constituents in the newly formed bone. Note the island of immature cartilage, arising within the synovium adjacent to the bone fragment.

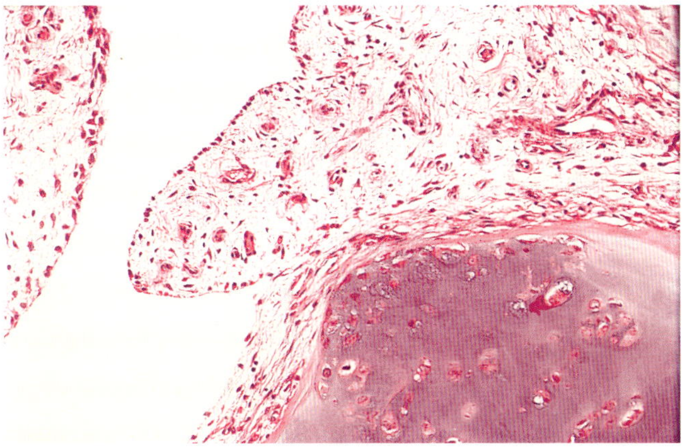

Figure 8-2. Synovial chondromatosis. The cartilage is formed within the synovium. Note the synovial epithelial lining surrounding the metaplastic cartilage fragment.

TABLE 8-1. Histology of Nodular and Diffuse Synovitis

Diffuse Synovitis (PVNS)	*Nodular Synovitis (GCTTS)*
Brown, bloody, villous	Yellow, nodular
Xanthoma cells	Xanthoma cells
Giant cells	Giant cells
Hemosiderin 3–4+	Hemosiderin ±
Villi	Circumscribed
Bone invasion 2+	Bone invasion ±

PVNS = pigmented villonodular synovitis; GCTTS = giant cell tumor of tendon sheath.

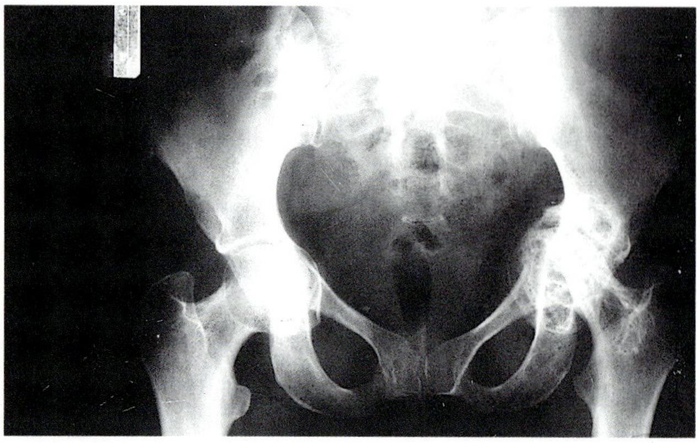

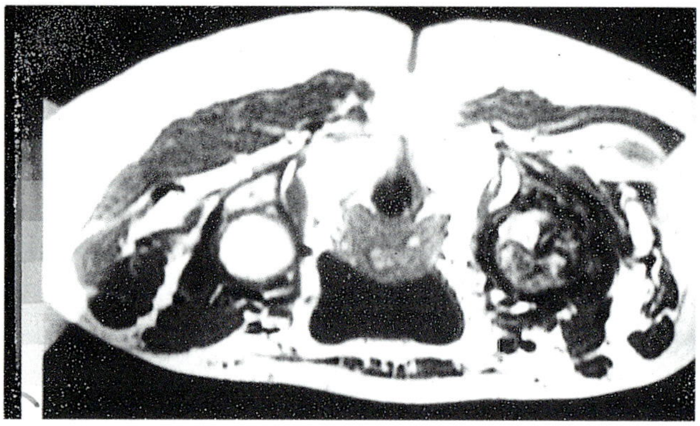

Figures 8-5, 8-6. Radiographic manifestations of pigmented villonodular synovitis. Note the extensive destruction of the head of the femur, with encroachment into the acetabulum. Pigmented villonodular synovitis will involve the entire synovium of a given joint, and because of its propensity to invade adjacent structures, will involve the acetabulum in the case of the hip, or both sides of the knee joint, or multiple bones in the ankle or foot. In this particular instance the only available therapy is total prosthesis.

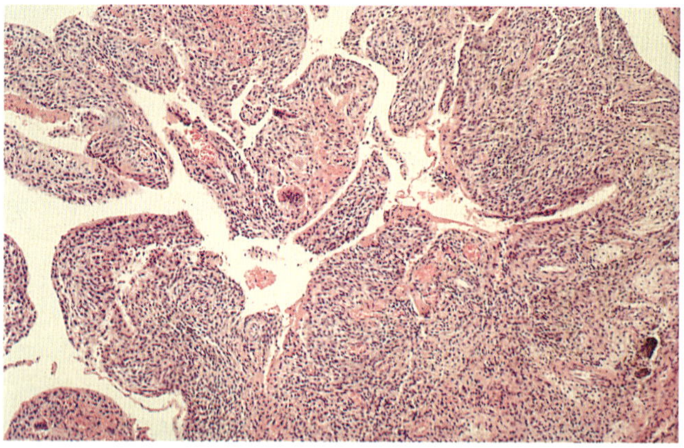

Figure 8-7. Pigmented villonodular synovitis. Note the extensive proliferation of the synovial tissue with an extremely cellular infiltrate replacing the normal stroma. Hemosiderin-laden macrophages, xanthomatous elements, giant cells, and residual connective tissue fibers are identified.

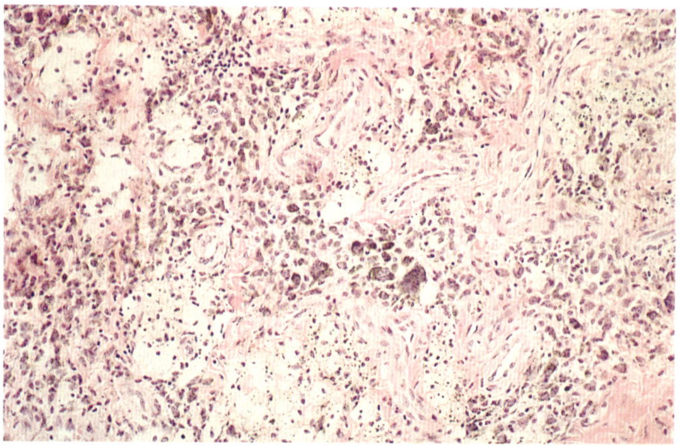

Figure 8-8. Giant cell tumor of tendon sheath. Numerous giant cells, xanthomatous elements, fibroblasts, and residual elements of tendon are the constituents of a giant cell tumor of tendon sheath or of a pigmented villonodular synovitis.

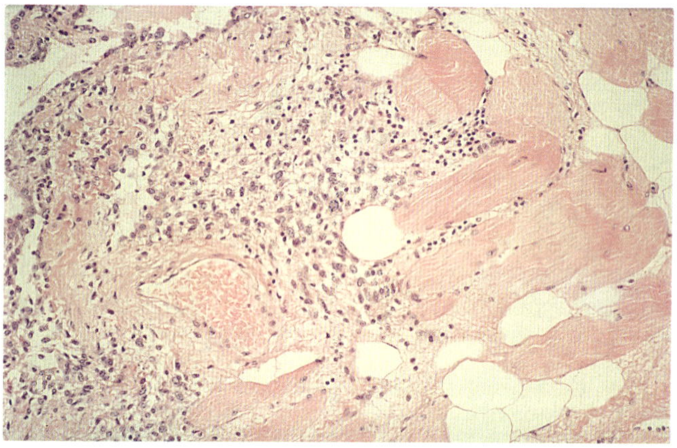

Figure 8-9. The aggressive nature of a pigmented villonodular synovitis is demonstrated by the invasion of the adjacent muscle tissue. Muscle, tendon, bone, and other articular structures are all engulfed in this process.

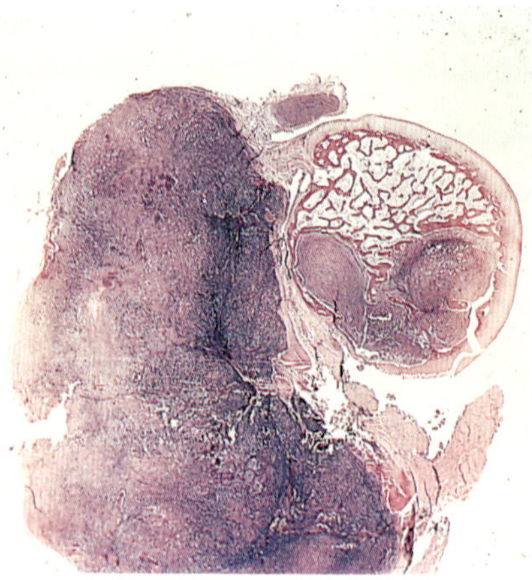

Figure 8-10. Nodular synovitis (giant cell tumor of tendon sheath), with a large soft tissue mass, but also involvement of the adjacent bone structure. From the viewpoint of histology, there is little if any discernible difference between the diffuse and the localized form, such as is seen in the small bones of the hands and feet.

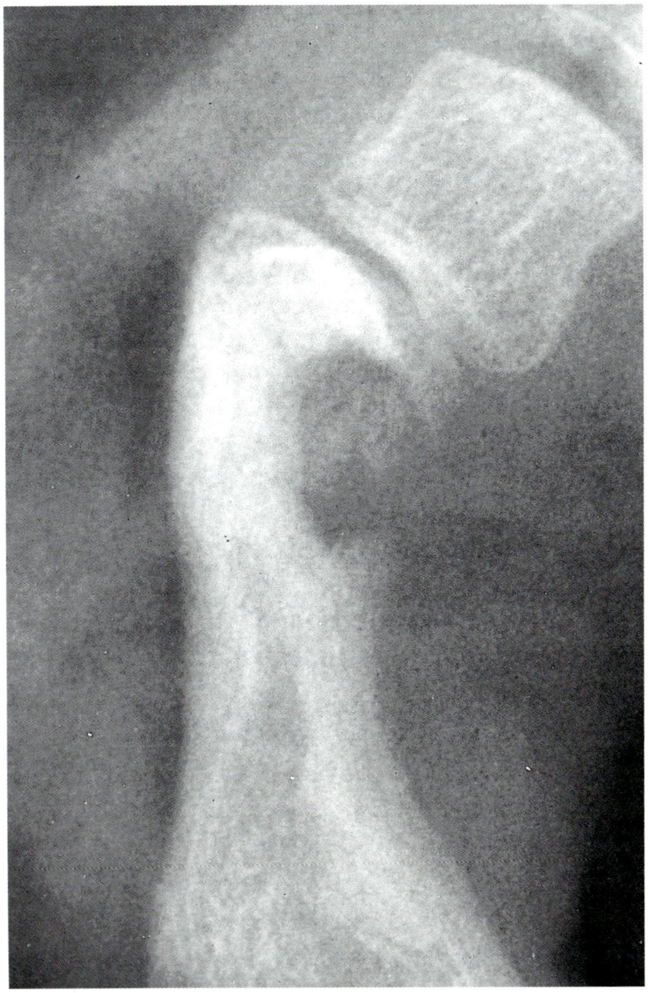

Figure 8-11. Radiographic manifestation of nodular synovitis invading the bone. Note the shape demarcation of the lesion, but no evidence of intraosseous expansion of bone. This is a clue that the lesion is entering the bone from the soft tissue, rather than extending into soft tissue from the bone itself.

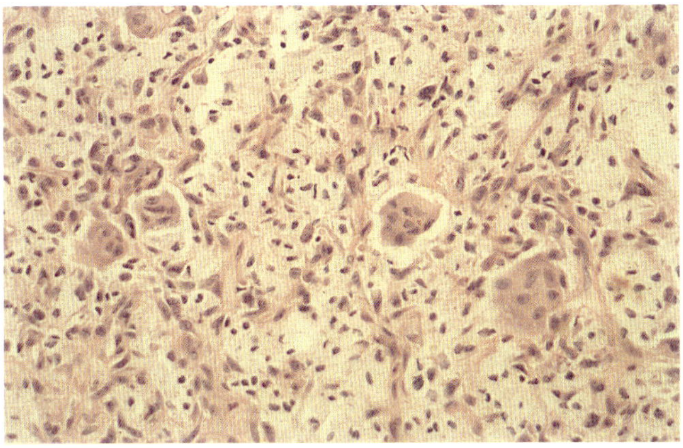

Figure 8-12. The histologic features of nodular synovitis are similar to diffuse synovitis.

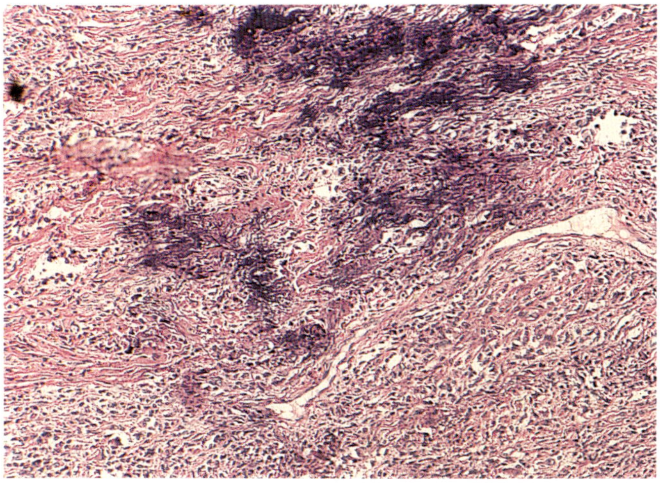

Figure 8-13. Occasionally nodular synovitis will exhibit foci of calcification. This calcification may be identified radiographically, but must be differentiated from the calcification often seen in a synovial sarcoma.

mas, fibrosarcomas, rhabdomyosarcomas, liposarcomas, and malignant fibrous histiocytomas of soft tissue.[19] The exact histologic diagnosis and differential diagnosis is a specialty unto itself and is not germane to this monograph. Treatment of all soft tissue tumors is basically similar and follows the principles laid down by Enneking.[20]

Synovial Sarcoma

The sarcoma which has its own particular history, characteristics, and distinct clinical course is the synovial sarcoma. Synovial sarcomas do not arise in joints, but rather in soft tissue at some distance from a joint. The tumor is characteristically composed of biphasic pattern: an epithelial as well as a spindled mesenchymal component. The epithelial component has certain histochemical characteristics which can be identified, particularly acid mucopolysaccharide production, and the spindle component may occasionally form collagen fibers. Although monophasic synovial sarcomas are de-

TABLE 8-2. Differential Diagnosis of Joint Lesions

1. Synovitis, nodular (localized, giant cell tumor of tendon sheath).
2. Diffuse, pigmented (pigmented villonodular synovitis).
3. Synovial chondromatosis.
4. Inflammatory synovial disease.
5. Fibroma of tendon sheath.

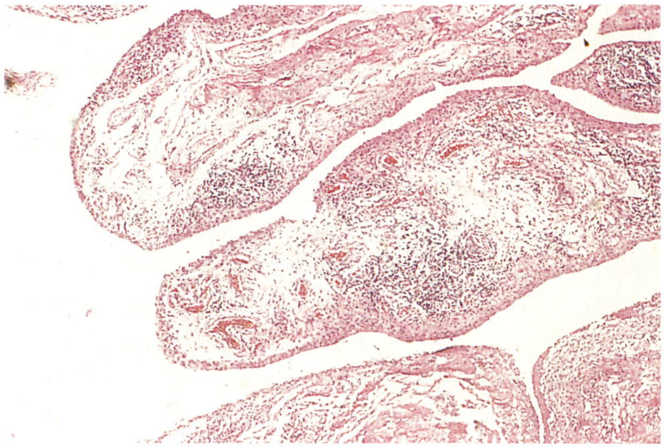

Figure 8-14. Proliferative synovitis. This type of synovial proliferation can exist with any inflammatory process, and should not be confused with pigmented villonodular synovitis, despite the presence of exaggerated villi. The response of the synovium to hemorrhage, trauma, or infection is similar, and consists of proliferation and accumulation of inflammatory cells within the villous structure.

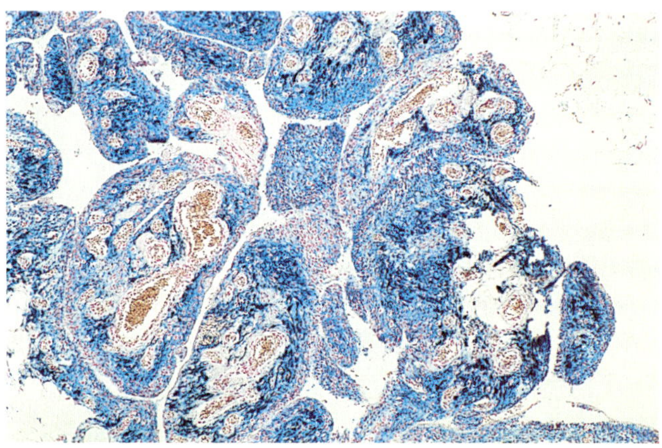

Figure 8-15. Hemorrhagic synovitis, secondary to trauma. Extensive hemosiderin deposition, as demonstrated by iron stains. There is no evidence of pigmented villonodular synovitis; these deposits are the breakdown products of bleeding within the articular space.

scribed in the literature,[21] the most common and reliable diagnostic feature is the biphasic pattern which must be searched for and is usually identifiable. The tumors may arise anywhere,[22] but most commonly involve the extremities, particularly the lower extremity. Approximately 30% of these patients have visible radiographic calcification at the time of presentation.[23]

Wide excision is the only appropriate therapy for this tumor. Prognosis depends upon tumor size. Five-year cures are not a measure of therapeutic effectiveness, since metastases occur after many years and 20-year intervals between primary and secondary metastases are not unknown.

Another distinct and unusual feature of this tumor is its tendency to metastasize to regional lymph nodes.

Synovial sarcoma should be considered whenever there is a soft tissue lesion composed of spindled cells. If the etiology is not clear, extensive sectioning should be performed to eliminate possible biphasic pattern. Soft tissue calcification is extremely suspicious for the presence of synovial sarcoma (Figures 8-16, 8-17).

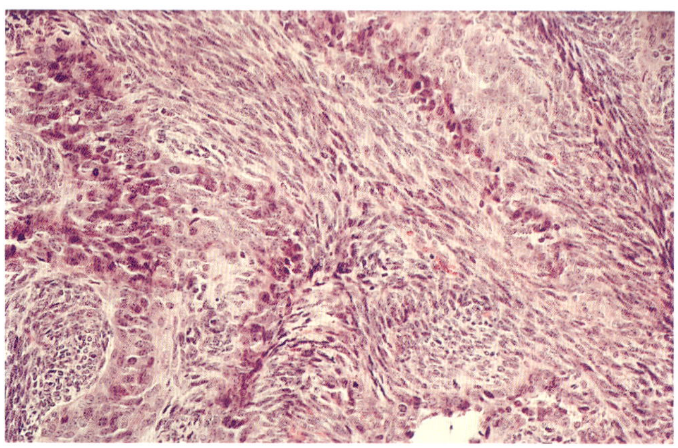

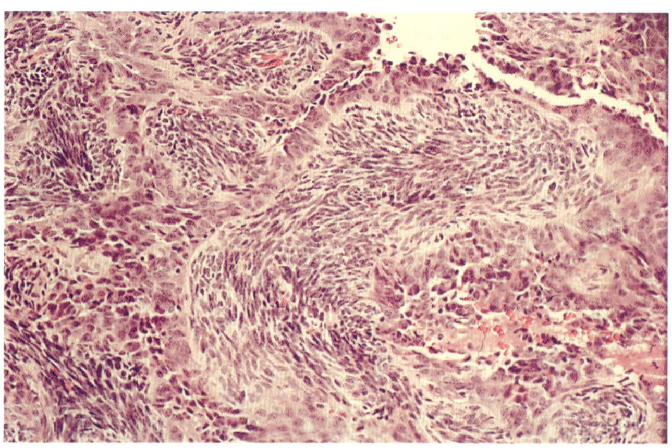

Figures 8-16, 8-17. Classical biphasic synovial sarcoma. Note the spindled and epithelioid components.

REFERENCES

1. Valmassy R, Ferguson H: Synovial osteochondromatosis. A brief review (Review). *J Am Podiatr Med Assoc* 82(8)427–431, 1992.
2. Bertoni F, Unni KK, Beabout JW, et al: Chondrosarcoma of the synovium. *Cancer* 67(1):155–162, 1991.
3. Kenan S, Abdelwahab IF, Klein MJ, et al: Case report 817: Synovial chondrosarcoma secondary to synovial chondromatosis (Review). *Skeletal Radiol* 22(8):623–626, 1993.
4. Ushijima M, Hashimoto H, Tsuneyoski M, et al: Giant cell tumor of tendon sheath (nodular tenosynovitis). A study of 207 cases to compare the large joint group with the common digit group. *Cancer* 57(4):875–884, 1989.
5. Wood GS, Backstead JH, Medeiros LJ, et al: The cells of giant cell tumor of tendon sheath resemble osteoclasts. *Am J Surg Pathol* 12:444–452, 1988.
6. Flandry F, Norwood LA: Pigmented villonodular synovitis of the shoulder. *Orthopedics* 12(5):715–718, 1989.
7. Karnezis TA, McMillan RD, Ivan C: Pigmented villonodular synovitis in a vertebra. *J Bone Joint Surg* 72:927, 1990.
8. Weidner N, Ghalla VR, Bonsib SM, et al: Giant cell tumors of synovium (pigmented villonodular synovitis) involving the vertebral column. *Cancer* 57:2030–2036, 1986.
9. Chung EB, Enzinger FM: Fibroma of tendon sheath. *Cancer* 44:1945–1954, 1979.
10. Weilbaecher TG, Rodriguez FH Jr: Fibroma of tendon sheath. *J Surg Oncology* 32:230–232, 1986.
11. Butt WP, Hardy G, Ostlere SJ: Pigmented villonodular synovitis of the knee: Computed tomographic appearance. *Skeletal Radiol* 19:191–206, 1990.
12. Jelinek JS, Kransdorf MJ, Utz JA, et al: Imaging of pigmented villonodular synovitis with emphasis on MR imaging. *Am J Roentgenol* 152:337–342, 1989.
13. Poletti SC, Gates HS, Martinez SM, et al: The use of magnetic resonance imaging in the diagnosis of pigmented villonodular synovitis. *Orthopedics* 13:185–190, 1990.
14. Ugai K, Kurosaka M, Hirohata K: Lipid microspherules in synovial fluid of patients with pigmented villonodular synovitis. *Arthritis Rheum* 31:1442–1446, 1988.
15. Dawiskiba S, Eriksson L, Elner A, et al: Diffuse pigmented villonodular synovitis of the temporomandibular joint diagnosed by fine needle aspiration cytology. *Diagn Cytopath* 5:301–304, 1989.
16. Bentley G, McAuliffe T: Pigmented villonodular synovitis. *Ann Rheum Dis* 49:210–211, 1990.
17. Schwartz HS, Unni KK, Pritchard DJ: Pigmented villonodular synovitis. A retrospective review of affected large joints. *Clin Orthop* 247:243–255, 1989.
18. Nielsen AL, Kiaer T: Malignant giant cell tumor of synovium and locally destructive pigmented villonodular synovitis: Ultrastructural and immunohistochemical study and review of the literature. *Hum Path* 20:765–771, 1989.
19. Kransdorf MJ, Meis JM: From the archives of the AFIP. Extraskeletal osseous and cartilaginous tumors of the extremities. *Radiographics* 13(4):853–884, 1993.
20. Enneking WF: *Musculoskeletal Tumor Surgery*. Vol 2. New York, Churchill Livingstone, 1983.
21. Dardick I, Ramjohn S, Thomas MJ, et al: Synovial sarcoma. Interrelationship of the biphasic and monophasic subtypes. *Pathol Res Pract* 187(7):871–885, 1991.
22. Fetsch JF, Meis JM: Synovial sarcoma of the abdominal wall. *Cancer* 72(2):469–477, 1993.
23. Michgrub S, Ghandur-Mnaymneh L, Dorfman HD, et al: Synovial sarcoma with extensive osteoid and bone formation. *Am J Surg Pathol* 17(4):357–363, 1993.

General References

Bullough PG: *Atlas of Orthopedic Pathology with Clinical and Radiologic Correlations,* ed. 2. New York, Gower Medical Publishing, 1992.

Campanacci M: *Bone and Soft Tissue Tumors.* New York, Springer-Verlag, 1990.

Fechner RE, Mills SE: Tumors of bone and cartilage. In: *Atlas of Tumor Pathology,* 3rd series, fasc 8. Washington, DC, Armed Forces Institute of Pathology 1993.

Huvos AG: *Bone Tumors: Diagnosis, Treatment, and Prognosis, ed. 2.* Philadelphia, WB Saunders, 1991.

Mirra JM, Picci R, Gold RH: *Bone Tumor. Clinical, Radiologic, and Pathologic Correlations.* Philadelphia, Lea and Febiger, 1989.

Resnick D, Niwayama G: *Diagnosis of Bone and Joint Disorders,* ed 2. Philadelphia, WB Saunders, 1988.

Schajowicz F: *Tumors and Tumorlike Lesions of Bone. Pathology, Radiology, and Treatment.* Berlin, Springer-Verlag 1994.

Schajowicz F: *WHO, International Histologic Classification of Tumours. Histologic Typing of Bone Tumours.* 1993.

Wold LE, McLeod RA, Sim FH, et al: *Atlas of Orthopedic Pathology.* Philadelphia, WB Saunders, 1990.

Index

Page numbers in italics refer to illustrations